Keto Diet

Cookbook

The Ultimate Guide for Women,
to Lose Weight Quickly
and Improve Health, with Appetizing
Recipes and Meal Plans

By
Anna Parker

reader acts of their own accord and releases the author and Publisher of any responsibility for the observance of tips, advice, counsel, strategies and techniques that may be offered in this volume.

Table of Contents

Introduction

Thank you for downloading the book, *"Keto for Women: The Ultimate Guide for Women to Lose Weight Quickly and Improve Health, with Appetizing Recipes and Meal Plans."*

This book contains proven information and strategies on getting the best out of the ketogenic diet for women.

The book targets the needs of women's bodies to help them achieve weight loss and other health benefits associated with the Keto diet. This book will guide you through your keto journey by helping you take the right amounts of carbs, proteins, and fats to help you with various health issues.

The book contains many keto recipes that are delicious and easy to make. There is also a 30-day meal plan for different caloric intake. Some other things covered in the book include:

- What is the Keto diet?
- Mistakes to Avoid on Keto Diet
- Foods to eat and avoid
- Weight loss on Keto…and many more.

Thanks once again for downloading this book. Enjoy reading and embracing the keto lifestyle.

To help me create more informative books like this, kindly leave a short review on Amazon. It's very important to me. Thank you.

Chapter 1: Keto Diet Explained

What is keto diet?

Ketogenic diet is a low-carb, high-fat, and adequate protein diet that burns fat to generate energy for the body. The maximum limit for carbohydrates is 50g per day.

Benefits of Keto Diet

Research has shown that the keto diet to be a great way to lose weight. That's cool and all, but losing weight shouldn't be the only thing you seek with a diet. You should have more energy and better indications of health, such as lower cholesterol. Starting a ketogenic diet can provide you with some amazing health benefits in addition to losing weight:

Prevention of diabetes: Diabetes is essentially an impaired function of insulin. The ketogenic diet is able to improve insulin sensitivity. Your body will require less insulin to lower blood glucose levels back to normal if there's a higher level of insulin sensitivity. The body doesn't burn fat when insulin levels are high. Therefore, it's important to improve insulin sensitivity levels to help better regulate blood glucose levels.

Lower Risk for Heart disease: Heart disease is one of the leading causes of death in the United States, and it includes many risk factors such as cholesterol levels, body

4

fat, blood sugar, and blood pressure. The ketogenic diet can help to improve these risk factors, thus lowering the risk of heart disease.

Getting rid of acne: Another cool side benefit is that it can help get rid of acne if you struggle with breakouts regularly. The ketogenic diet will help to lower insulin levels by eating less processed foods and sugar, which can help prevent acne.

Cancer treatment: The ketogenic diet is currently being used to treat several different types of cancer, and it can slow tumor growth. Of course, there is a need for more research for conclusive evidence.

Increase HDL cholesterol levels: There are two different kinds of cholesterol—HDL, which stands for high-density lipoproteins and LDL, which stands for low-density lipoproteins. Your HDL is the good cholesterol that you want to increase because it's responsible for carrying cholesterol to the liver to be excreted or reused. LDL's on the other hand, are bad cholesterol and are responsible for carrying cholesterol away from the liver and into the body. Research shows one of the best ways to increase your HDL level is to increase your fat intake. You'll easily be able to achieve that with the standard ketogenic protocol of 75% of your calories coming from fat.

Lower blood pressure: Lowering your carbohydrate intake has been shown to decrease hypertension. Having higher blood pressure increases your risk of developing diseases such as heart disease and stroke.

Decrease triglyceride levels: Triglycerides are a fat molecule. It might sound counter-intuitive that increasing your fat intake would decrease the number of triglycerides in the blood, but it really does. This occurs because carbs are one of the biggest contributors to increasing triglycerides. Therefore, by decreasing carb intake, you'll decrease the number of triglycerides in your blood.

More weight loss than a typical diet: restricting calories on a keto diet helps in losing weight. People restricting calories on a keto diet lose weight faster than individuals restricting calories on a low-fat diet. The main reason for this is because low-carb diets lower insulin levels, which will cause the body to get rid of excess sodium within the first few weeks of starting the diet.

A positive way to lose your appetite: When you go on a diet and restrict your calories, you start to feel hungry. If your feelings of hunger start to get out of control, you're more likely to quit and give up on your diet—and obviously, if you quit and go back to your old habits, you have no chance of losing weight and improving your health. Luckily, eating a low-carb diet has been shown to decrease appetite. This is critical because it'll allow you to lower your overall caloric intake without having to worry about getting extra hungry.

Health

There are many health conditions that either uniquely affect women or affect women more frequently than men. The keto diet helps with several of them, which we'll briefly explore here.

Polycystic Ovary Syndrome (PCOS)

Polycystic ovary syndrome (PCOS), which is among endocrine disorders that are very common, is said to be caused by hormone imbalance. According to Medscape, roughly 4 to 12 percent of women have PCOS, but many don't even know it. Symptoms include excessive hair growth, irregular periods, difficulty getting pregnant, and high blood sugar. Scientists still do not know exactly what causes PCOS, but the accepted theory is that it results from a mixture of lifestyle and genetics. A 2005 study found that when obese women with PCOS were placed on a keto diet for 24 days, their body weights decreased by 17 percent, testosterone levels lowered by 22 percent, and fasting insulin levels saw a 54 percent decrease. In 2017, another study showed that the keto diet reduced circulating insulin levels, which improved hormonal imbalances and resumed ovulation, resulting in improved pregnancy rates.

Endometriosis and Uterine Fibroids

You've probably heard of endometriosis, even if you have no idea what it is. It is yet another condition that affects women, and it occurs when the uterine lining, normally found inside of your uterus, grows outside of your uterus. According to Medscape, it occurs in about 6 percent to 10 percent of women in the United States. Symptoms of endometriosis include abdominal pain, heavy periods, and infertility. Although doctors have not identified a cause, genetics may play a role. Some theories suggest endometriosis might be an autoimmune condition or could be related to high estrogen levels. The same is true of uterine fibroids. Many physicians believe that an environment of high insulin and estrogen in a woman's body may contribute to fibroid growth as well as endometriosis, so, again, the lower insulin levels achieved on a keto diet could help.

Autoimmune Conditions

Autoimmune conditions are more prevalent in women than in men by a factor of two to one. There are 80—yes, 80—autoimmune conditions that result in your immune system mistakenly attacking either a part of your body or your whole body, as with lupus. Autoimmune conditions and diseases have been on the rise over the past couple of decades, and some scientists believe that high sugar and highly processed foods increase inflammation, which might set off autoimmune responses. According to Jeff Volek, Ph.D., RD, the chief science officer at Virta Health, the keto diet has been shown to decrease inflammation and could help in the treatment of autoimmune conditions. These benefits are still being researched, so if you have an autoimmune condition, ask your doctor's opinion about going keto.

Thyroid Conditions

Oh, guess what?! Women are also more likely to experience thyroid dysfunction compared to men. Luckily the keto diet can be beneficial for thyroid conditions. When done correctly, eating keto stabilizes blood sugar levels, which allows for a balanced production of thyroid hormones. This is much better for your body than the roller-coaster effect that the typical American diet has on blood sugar.

The Nutritional Needs of Women

It's probably not news to you that women have unique physiology and thus have different nutritional needs from men. First and foremost, our calorie needs are different. Men generally have larger bodies, greater muscle mass, and a need for more calories. Even a man with the same height and weight as his female counterpart will burn roughly 400 more calories per day than she will. Lucky us, right?

Beyond that, it has been well established that we need more vitamins and minerals due to hormonal changes, menstruation, and childbearing. The most vital include calcium, vitamin D, a vitamin B complex, iron, iodine, and magnesium. These are notoriously difficult to obtain in adequate amounts on a calorie-restricted diet. Thankfully the keto diet is no such thing, which is why it's better for your body.

Here are some of the vitamins and minerals that are plentiful on the keto diet.

CALCIUM

Women are more prone to osteoporosis compared to men, which increases the risk of fractures. Foods rich in calcium that are keto staples include full-fat dairy products, sardines, salmon, and kale.

VITAMIN D

From helping the body absorb calcium and building stronger bones to decreasing inflammation, vitamin D has been dubbed a miracle cure by many. While the best way to get it is by going outside and soaking up those sun rays, you can also eat plenty of fatty fish, egg yolks, mushrooms, and animal liver—all foods that are emphasized on the keto diet!

B VITAMINS

The entire B complex includes B1, B2, B3, B5, B6, B9, B12, and biotin, which are water-soluble essential nutrients. When you think of B9, also known as folate, think green. High-folate foods include spinach, collard greens, mustard greens, asparagus, broccoli, and avocado. B12 is generally found naturally in animal products, including fish, meat, poultry, eggs, and milk.

IRON

This mineral helps with red blood cell formation, wound healing, immune function, and energy production. Women are often iron-deficient due to blood loss during their menstrual cycles. Iron can be found in keto-friendly foods such as red meats, liver, and poultry.

IODINE

This mineral is crucial for healthy fetus development during pregnancy. Keto-approved foods that are high in iodine include seafood, seaweed, eggs, and iodized salt.

MAGNESIUM

This is a mineral that affects more than 300 enzyme systems in a woman's body and regulates biochemical reactions, including protein synthesis, nerve regeneration, blood sugar control, and blood pressure regulation. Foods with magnesium levels include all leafy greens and avocado.

As you can see, the keto diet contains foods with essential nutrients specific to the needs of a woman's body, so you don't need to worry about creating a vitamin or mineral deficiency by eating this way.

Why Starting a New Diet Can Be Hard

Changing the way you eat is hard. At the beginning of any diet, you have to override cravings for things your body has grown to expect you will eat.

The keto diet is a regimen that may initially feel even more challenging because it flies in the face of so many nutritional dicta you've probably been taught since grade school. Although the diet has gained popularity, there are many critics who will try to dissuade you from even starting. The best thing is to do your own research. Knowing how and why this diet works is just as important as knowing what to eat.

Among the common mistakes made by women when starting the keto diet is not eating enough calories from fat. Eating healthy fat will send signals to your body that there is an abundance of food available. This message means your body will not dive into metabolic conservation mode as it does when there is a caloric deficit. Eating healthy fat also gives you a psychological boost. Being able to eat rich foods and feeling satisfied rather than starving yourself on low-calorie cakes is a gift, as far as I'm concerned. This satisfaction will motivate you to stay on this diet and reap all of its benefits.

How the Ketogenic Diet Works

As you're aware, fuel is necessary to power us through everything from sleeping to exercise, and we get this fuel from food. But you may not be aware that there are two sources of this fuel: We can get it from glucose (from carbohydrates) or from fatty acids (from fats). The fuel your body uses is mostly determined by the composition of your diet. When eating a high-carbohydrate diet (you know, full of processed flours, bread, pasta, whole grains, root veggies, and tropical fruits—aka the standard American diet), your body will break this food down into simple sugars called glucose.

In both men and women, glucose is the default fuel. When eating carbohydrates, especially in their refined forms such as bread and pasta, your insulin rapidly increases. This lets the taking up of glucose by your muscles and brain for energy. Any excess glucose is then stored as glycogen in your liver. Roughly 6 to 24 hours after a meal, your insulin levels fall, and the glycogen stored in your liver releases glucose to keep blood sugar levels steady. Several hours later, if you still have not eaten, gluconeogenesis, the breakdown of protein, occurs to provide some energy. Now, if you still have not eaten for one or two days, or you have taken in minimal sugar, your body starts searching for another fuel source: fat. The process of breaking down fat for fuel is called ketosis.

What Is Ketosis?

Ketosis is a normal process that our bodies undergo. Even if you're not trying to reach ketosis, you may very well have experienced a mild form of it if you ever have skipped a meal or exercised for more than an hour, or simply did not eat carbohydrates one day. Whenever your energy needs increase, and there aren't enough incoming carbohydrates, your body uses fat to produce that energy. This process is a natural part of life from an evolutionary point of view. Our bodies have evolved to deal with food scarcity. The keto diet works by naturally changing your metabolism to your advantage.

Who cannot Use Keto diet?

If you have Type 1 Diabetes, you should not use the Keto diet. Due to the process by which the Keto diet lowers your carb intake, it can cause your blood sugar to decrease. This can be symptomatic for those suffering from Type 1

Diabetes. When your blood sugar reduces, it can cause hypoglycemia. If you are on insulin or insulin-lowering drugs, check with your doctor about the Keto diet before trying it. Sometimes, you can speak with your doctor about the Keto diet, and they will reduce your insulin shots or medications. With that, you can participate in the keto diet to get healthy.

If you are someone that suffers from adrenal and thyroid issues, you should approach the Keto diet with caution. People that suffer from this condition do not handle stress very well. So, this could be more problematic than helpful. Ketosis can cause your body some stress, and this would essentially be difficult because of your thyroid or adrenal gland illness.

Children are not a good fit for the Keto diet. Because they are still growing and need adequate nutrition daily, this should not be tried on anyone under the age of 18.

People who are underweight and undernourished should not try the Keto diet. If your BMI is 18 kg/m2 or less, it is not recommended that you limit your intake of calories. This can lead to malnourishment.

Pregnant or breastfeeding moms should not use the Keto diet. With breastfeeding, you need to have all the nutrients you can. So, to limit your options of food intake would cause undue harm to yourself and your baby.

Macros Calculation
Twinkie diet

Twinkie Diet refers to an experiment conducted a few years ago at Kansas State University by Mark Haub, a professor of nutrition. Mark Haub wanted to discredit the claim of many diets' specialists, arguing that calorie-counting is totally unimportant and not useful for weight-loss. Haub wasn't claiming that eating junk-food (cream cakes, cookies, chips, snacks) has benefits to our bodies, but he is demonstrating that it is possible to lose weight when the Calories are deficient, regardless of the quality of what a person eats.

Mark Haub was limited to an intake of 1800 Calories a day while his daily requirements are about 2600 Calories, which made a daily caloric deficit of 800 Calories.

At the end of the experiment, Mark Haub lost weight as he expected. His bodyweight went to 174 from 207 pounds. The body mass index (BMI) dropped to 24.9 from 28.8.

The LDL decreased by 20%

The HDL rose by 20%

The triglycerides (a type of fat (lipid) found in the blood) decreased by 39%.

The body fat went down to 24.9% from 33.4%

The main conclusion of the experiment is obvious: the caloric deficit works. However, we have to notice that calories are not equal. You have to choose high-quality food by following the guidelines about choosing, carbohydrates, fats, and protein.

Calculation of the total daily energy expenditure

The calculation of your keto diet macros begins by establishing your TDEE (total daily energy expenditure) and setting a Calorie Deficit

You should start by setting a Calorie deficit target before you calculate your ketogenic macros. 10% is a safe point for starting.

Take this example to bring clarity to the calculation method. A moderately active woman, Cherry, who is 30 years old, 5'5", and 180 pounds, will need 2120 Calories per day. That represents her total daily energy expenditure (TDEE).

Calculation of the WLTDE (Weight Loss TDEE) and Calorie deficit

In a 10% Calorie deficit plan, the Weight Loss TDEE (WLTDE) is 1908 Calories. This is calculated by multiplying 90% by her TDEE (2120 Calories) = 1908 Calories.

The calorie deficit equals 212 Calories per day. This is calculated by multiplying 10% by the TDEE (2120 Calories) = 212 Calories.

At this stade, Cherry can expect to have 1484 Calories deficit per week. This is calculated by multiplying 7 (days) by her daily Calorie deficit (212 Calories) = 1484 Calories.

She can expect to lose 0.424 pounds per week. This is calculated by dividing the Calorie deficit per week (1484) by 3500, which represents a loss of one pound.

Calculation of the Carbohydrates Quantity?

The ketogenic diet is a low-carb diet, and your daily carbohydrates intake must represent 5% of your total daily intake. That means that 5% of your total Calories must come from carbs. For the majority of people, this represents 20 to 30 grams of carbohydrate per day.

Let us pursue our example:

YOUR NORMAL TDEE= 2120 Calories (This is what the woman' body will burn normally)

HER CALORIE DEFICIT= 212 Calories (10%)

HER WEIGHT LOSS TDEE =2120 - 212 = 1908 Calories (what she will eat)

How to calculate the number of carbohydrates?

The woman weight loss TDEE is 1.908, 5% of carbs means you should only consume 23.85 g per day. This is calculated by multiplying 5% by 1680 = 95.4. Then divide

95.4 by four because there are four calories per gram of carbs.

Calculation of the Proteins Quantity?

Some people on a ketogenic diet make a mistake and consume too much protein.

Your body will convert protein to energy for the body and prevent your body from burning extra fat, which is counterproductive. So, to take the maximum advantage of the ketogenic diet, you must limit your daily intake in protein to 20%.

Protein should come mainly from animal meats, full-fat dairy, eggs, and whole food sources.

That means that 20% of your total Calories must come from protein.

Let us pursue our example:

The woman weight loss TDEE is 1.908. 20 % of protein means she should only consume 95,4 g per day. This is calculated by multiplying 20% by 1908 = 381,6. Then divide 381,6 by four because there are four calories per gram of protein.

Calculation of the Fat Quantity?

The rest of your remaining daily Calories, i.e., 75% daily calories should come from fat.

It's essential that you eat healthy sources of fat and avoid processed fats and some vegetable oils.

The woman weight loss TDEE is 1.908, 75% of fat means she should consume 159 g per day. This is calculated by multiplying 75% by 1908 = 1431. Then divide 1,431 by nine because there are nine calories per gram of fat.

So, for a moderately active woman, aged 30 years old, 5'5", 180 pounds with a weight loss TDEE of 1908 Calories. The keto macros are:

Protein: 95,4 grams (20%)

Fat: 159 grams (75%)

Carbs: 23.85 grams (5%)

Once you gain a better insight and understanding of your individual macronutrient breakdown and keep tracking your Keto macros, you'll see how fast you start to achieve your weight-loss goal.

Additionally, counting your Keto macronutrients will enable you to enter Ketosis much faster.

For more convenience you can use the Keto Calculator in this URL address:

https://calculo.io/keto-calculator

Problems You May Have Using Keto

Fast muscle catabolism: This process literally happens overnight when you restrict carbohydrates. You see, without carbohydrates, your body turns to its own tissues for energy. In other words, you put your muscle tissue on the dinner plate.

Negative hormone production: High protein eating translates into more cortisol being released into your body. And not only does cortisol break down muscle protein, but it also decreases immunity.

Less mental performance: You see, although your body can convert muscle protein to sugar for your brain, it is not a very efficient process. Subsequently, your mental performance decreases. Therefore, if you need to maintain mental performance, high protein diets are probably not for you.

Gloomy moods: Certain neurotransmitters in your brain need carbs to replenish themselves. Therefore, if you stop eating carbs, your mood deteriorates. This is among the key reasons why fitness professionals suffer from extreme mood swings when restricting carbs

Less intensity: For the absolute best workouts, your body needs full levels of muscle carbohydrates. Without them, you cannot reach your intensity potential. This, in turn, decreases the number of calories your body burns outside of your workouts.

Ketogenic Diet and Fertility: If the priority is getting pregnant and you get into the ketogenic abruptly, your body may understand that this is not the time to get pregnant, and you stop menstruating.

This does not mean that ketogenic causes infertility. In contrast, women with polycystic ovaries even menstruate again and improve fertility with this lifestyle, as it improves insulin resistance.

It's all a matter of individualizing and understanding that your body can respond this way (not a rule). If it happens, I'll give you some tips to improve and start over differently to make it work for you!

A low-calorie diet or excessive weight loss with a sharp drop in body fat percentage (<8-9%) can have the same effect. In this case, only weight gain solves the problem.

This occurs on any low carb diet (low carb or not) that results in excessive loss of body fat.

Loss of definition: You need carbohydrates to have a toned look. You see, carbs pull water into your muscles. If you stop eating them, your muscles dehydrate and end up looking like deflated balloons. So be conscious of this before avoiding carbs.

High protein diets are not all their cracked up to be. You see, although they do cause very rapid short-term water weight loss, they are not very good for your health.

Chapter 2: Common Mistakes to Avoid

Do you feel like you are giving your all to the keto diet, but you still aren't seeing the results you want? You are measuring ketones, working out, and counting your macros, but you still aren't losing the weight you want. Here are the most common mistakes that most people make when beginning the keto diet.

Too Many Snacks

There are many snacks you can enjoy while following the keto diet, like nuts, avocado, seeds, and cheese. But snacking can be an easy way to get too many calories into the diet while giving your body an easy fuel source besides stored fat. Snacks need to be only used if you frequently hunger between meals. If you aren't extremely hungry, let your body turn to your stored fat for its fuel between meals instead of dietary fat.

Not Consuming Enough Fat

The ketogenic diet isn't all about low carbs. It's also about high fats. You need to be getting about 75 percent of your calories from healthy fats, five percent from carbs, and 20 percent from protein. Fat makes you feel fuller longer, so if you eat the correct amount, you will minimize your carb cravings, and this will help you stay in ketosis. This will help your body burn fat faster.

Consuming Excessive Calories

You may hear people say you can eat what you want on the keto diet as long as it is high in fat. Even though we want that to be true, it is very misleading. Healthy fats need to make up the biggest part of your diet. If you eat more calories than what you are burning, you will gain weight, no matter what you eat, because these excess calories get stored as fat. An average adult only needs about 2,000 calories each day, but this will vary based on many factors like activity level, height, and gender.

Consuming a lot of Dairies

For many people, dairy can cause inflammation and keeps them from losing weight. Dairy is a combo food meaning it has carbs, protein, and fats. If you eat a lot of cheese as a snack for the fat content, you are also getting a dose of carbs and protein with that fat. Many people can tolerate dairy, but moderation is the key. Remember to factor in the protein content.

Consuming a lot of Protein

The biggest mistake that most people make when just beginning the keto diet is consuming too much protein. Excess protein gets converted into glucose in the body called gluconeogenesis. This is a natural process where the body converts the energy from fats and proteins into glucose when glucose isn't available. When following a ketogenic diet, gluconeogenesis happens at different rates to keep body function. Our bodies don't need a lot of carbs, but we do need glucose. You can eat absolute zero carbs, and through gluconeogenesis, your body will convert other substances into glucose to be used as fuel. This is why carbs only make up five percent of your macros. Some parts of our bodies need carbs to survive, like kidney, medulla, and red blood cells. With gluconeogenesis, our bodies make and stores extra glucose as glycogen just in case supplies become too low.

In a normal diet, when carbs are always available, gluconeogenesis happens slowly because the need for glucose is extremely low. Our body runs on glucose and will store excess protein and carbs as fat.

It does take time for our bodies to switch from using glucose to burning fats. Once you are in ketosis, the body will use fat as the main fuel source and will start to store excess protein as glycogen.

Not Getting Enough Water

Water is crucial for your body. Water is needed for all your body does, and this includes burning fat. If you don't drink enough water, it can cause your metabolism to slow down, and this can halt your weight loss. Drinking 64 ounces or one-half gallon every day will help your body burn fat, flush out toxins, and circulate nutrients. When you are just beginning the keto diet, you might need to drink more water since your body will begin to get rid of body fat by flushing it out through urine.

Consuming Too Many Sweets

Some people might indulge in keto brownies and keto cookies that are full of sugar substitutes just because their net carb content is low, but you have to remember that you are still eating calories. Eating sweets might increase your carb cravings. Keto sweets are great on occasion; they don't need to be a staple in the diet.

Not Getting Enough Sleep

Getting plenty of sleep is needed in order to lose weight effectively. Without the right amount of sleep, your body will feel stressed, and this could result in your metabolism slowing down. It might cause it to store fat instead of burning fat. When you feel tired, you are more tempted to drink more lattes for energy, eat a snack to give you an extra boost, or order takeout rather than cooking a healthy meal. 7-9 hours of sleep are enough. Understand that your body uses that time to burn fat without you even lifting a finger.

Low on Electrolytes

Most people will experience the keto flu when you begin this diet. This happens for two reasons when your body changes from burning carbs to burning fat, your brain might not have enough energy, and this, in turn, can cause grogginess, headaches, and nausea. You could be dehydrated, and your electrolytes might be low since the keto diet causes you to urinate often.

Getting the keto flu is a great sign that you are heading in the right direction. You can lessen these symptoms by drinking more water or taking supplements that will balance your electrolytes.

Consuming Hidden Carbs

Many foods look like they are low carb, but they aren't. You can find carbs in salad dressings, sauces, and condiments. Be sure to check nutrition labels before you try new foods to make sure it doesn't have any hidden sugar or carbs. It takes less than half a minute to skim the label, and it might be the difference between whether or not you'll lose weight.

If you have successfully ruled out all of the above, but you still aren't losing weight, you might need to talk with your doctor to make sure you don't have any health problems that could be preventing your weight loss. This is tough, but stick with it, stay positive, and stay in the game. When the keto diet is done correctly, it is one of the best ways to lose weight.

Chapter 3: Foods to Eat Keto

Healthy Fats

- Saturated (goose fat, tallow, clarified butter / ghee, coconut oil, duck fat, lard, butter, chicken fat)
- Monounsaturated (olive, macadamia, and avocado oil)
- Polyunsaturated omega 3s (seafood and fatty fish)

Non-starchy vegetables

- Spinach
- Endive
- Bamboo Shoots
- Asparagus
- Lettuce
- Cucumber
- Kale
- Radishes
- Celery Stalk
- Chives
- Zucchini

Fruits, e.g., avocado, berries

Nuts and seeds

Macadamia nuts, pine nuts, walnuts, sunflower seeds, sesame seeds, hemp seeds, pumpkin seeds, pecans, hazelnuts, almonds

Dairy Products
Cream cheese
Heavy whipping cream
Whole milk yogurt (unsweetened)

Beverages

- Water
- Unsweetened herbal tea
- Unsweetened coconut milk
- Decaf coffee
- Unsweetened almond milk
- Unsweetened soy milk
- Unsweetened herbal tea

Protein

Fish: cod, halibut, tuna, salmon, trout, flounder, mackerel, snapper, and catfish.

Meat: Goat, Beef, Lamb, and other wild game

Poultry: Chicken meat, duck meat, and quail meat

Shellfish: Squid, Clams, scallops, lobster, mussels, crab, and oysters,

Whole Eggs

Pork products

Sausage and bacon

Peanut Butter

Dressings

- Balsamic Vinegar
- Ranch
- Blue Cheese
- Apple Cider Vinegar
- Creamy Caesar

Spices

- Oregano
- Black Pepper
- Rosemary
- Basil
- Thyme
- Sea salt
- Cumin
- Parsley
- Sage
- Cayenne Pepper

Chapter 4: Foods to Avoid

To reach ketosis successfully, do your best to prevent and rid your body of foods that will hold you back from your goal. Most foods to avoid are high in carbohydrates and do not allow your body to burn fat for energy. You should avoid these foods:

Root Vegetables

Vegetables that grow and get pulled from the ground are high in carbohydrates and take you away from ketosis. Such vegetables include potatoes, beets, radishes, carrots, onions, and parsnips.

Sweet Fruits

While following the ketogenic diet, you should avoid most fruits. Fruits contain fructose (similar to glucose) and are bad for reaching ketosis. Not only avoid fruits; stay away from products made with fresh fruit, such as juices and extracts. If you eat fruits, then keep it in moderation.

Grains

Obviously, avoid all foods made with processed grains. Grains contain additives that can negatively affect your insulin levels. Such grains include bread, pasta, cakes, breadcrumbs, cookies, and pastries.

Diet Soda

Diet soda claims not to contain sugars or carbs; it contains artificial sweeteners equally as detrimental as regular sugar. Artificial sweeteners enhance your carbohydrate intake and prevent you from reaching the metabolic state of ketosis.

Alcohol

Most alcohol beverages consist of none, or low carbs, but can still be bad for a keto lifestyle. Alcohol prevents the fat burning process or dramatically slows it down, because your body will need to process the alcohol first before the fat. To be successful with this diet, limit your alcohol intake.

Processed Foods

Avoid processed or packaged foods. Such foods are packed with artificial additives that can stray you from ketosis. Instead of choosing processed foods, pick organic and real ingredients.

Opinions differ between some individuals and sources, but you get the concept. The ketogenic diet and instant pot have plenty of lot in common. It can be used together to make fast, tasty, and healthy dishes that will improve your life. Since the keto diet asks you to avoid greasy foods, the instant pot helps by softening up foods using pressure and heat. With that being said, let's use the instant pot to prepare ketogenic meals for better health.

Chapter 5: Tips for the Keto Journey

To achieve success with your keto diet, here are some practical tips that you have to follow:

Lower carb consumption

Since the keto diet is a low carb diet, obviously, you need to reduce your consumption of carbohydrates. This is the key that will help you achieve ketosis.

This can be a big challenge at first, especially if you are used to including carbs in your daily diet. However, you can gradually remove carbs from your diet to help your body reach the state of ketosis.

It is imperative that you limit your carb consumption to 20 to 50 net grams per day.

Consume coconut oil

Experts say that consuming coconut oil can help your body achieve natural ketosis more quickly. This is because coconut oil contains medium-chain triglycerides that are absorbed by the body rapidly and immediately converted into ketones.

Just make sure that you slowly add coconut oil to your diet to avoid side effects such as diarrhea and stomach cramps. Start by taking in only one teaspoon per day for one week. Increase intake to two tablespoons each day in the second week.

Increase physical activity

Anyone who's using the ketogenic diet should know that just like with any other weight loss diet program, diet is not effective on its own. You also need to get moving and to engage in regular exercise. If you are more active, it will be easier for your body to reach ketosis. Exercise increases ketone levels, and should, therefore, be included in your weight loss regimen.

Focus on consuming healthy fats

While it's true that unhealthy fats are not completely restricted in the ketogenic diet, it would still be a good idea to focus more on consuming healthy fats.

Healthy fats include avocado oil, coconut oil, olive oil, tallow, and lard.

Take sufficient amount of protein

Some keto dieters make the mistake of focusing only on the consumption of carbs and fat, forgetting about the equally important nutrient, which is protein.

But in order for you to maximize the ketone levels, it is important to take in enough protein so that the liver will receive a sufficient number of amino acids that the body needs to burn fat and lose weight.

Measure ketone levels

If you are not sure whether you've reached ketosis or not, you should make use of a ketone meter, which can be purchased in drugstores. There are testers that measure ketones in the breath, urine, and blood. The one that measures ketones in the blood is the most accurate but also the most expensive.

Be determined and consistent

As with any other diet program, you need to have both determination and consistency to achieve your goals with the ketogenic diet program. You cannot reach your weight loss objectives if you are not determined to succeed and if you are not consistent in following the diet's strict rules.

Chapter 6: Ketogenic Diet and Weight-Loss

Ketogenic diet enables the breaking down of unwanted fats and stored substances by the body. It is one of the main bodybuilding solutions which helps in lowering fat content in the body while creating muscle. Many of the bodybuilders on the keto diet regime set their everyday calorie intake to 20% more than their typical calorie level. The figure is not set, but individuals adjust it accordingly. It is not a set figure but a guide and could be adjusted on an individual basis.

It is advised loading up on carbs for a three-day cycle while on the keto plan. Eat about 1000 calories of carbs on the third day a couple of hours before exercising. For carb loading, there are two options;

    i. eating what you like.

    ii. start with carbs with higher glycemic and then going to the lower ones.

Carb loading is good for an intense workout because it enables endurance by enhancing glycogen in the muscles.

For instance, let us say you start off carb-loading on Friday. By Sunday, your muscle tissues will have a substantial amount of glycogen in them. This is the day you ought to exercise. It is optimal to only work out half of the body at this time with weights. Schedule your next exercise routine on Wednesday, and be sure to consume 1000 calories worth of carbs prior to your routine. By Wednesday, your glycogen levels will likely be low, but the pre-workout carb load will allow you to work out intensely. You will now do exercises that target the other half of your body.

The next exercise session should be scheduled for Friday at the beginning of the three-day cycle of loading up on carbohydrates. This training session has to be a complete overall body workout with 1-2 sets per workout completed until failure. Make barbell rows, bench presses, military presses, barbell/dumbbell curls, triceps pushdowns, squats, lunges, deadlifts, and reverse curls the focus of your training. The aim is to deplete your glycogen stores within the body completely. Nevertheless, keep cardio to a minimum. Ten-minute warm-ups in advance of each workout are fine but do not go overboard.

Why It's Tougher for Women to Lose Weight

Have you noticed that men lose weight faster than women? You may wonder why you would begin a weight loss program with a man, do the same exercise routine, use similar calorie goals, and at the end of the day, he would shed more weight than you and even do it quickly.

This isn't fair, but a man's body and that of a woman are different. Below are some of the reasons men tend to shed weight quicker, and what the obstacles could be.

Evolutionary makeup.

A woman has the tendency to get pregnant, and her body is designed to have about ten percent fats more than a male counterpart. The same can be said for muscle mass.

As a result of the fact that muscles burn a lot of calories, the male counterparts have a metabolism rate that's higher. What this translates to is that men can easily shed their calories faster than women.

Undiagnosed PCOS, or polycystic ovary syndrome.

This is one endocrine disorder that's common in about ten percent of women, but only about thirty percent of them know about their status. When a lady has this, she tends to experience irregular periods, great weight gain, insulin resistance, as well as the risk of being obese.

Menopause

Only women go through menopause, and the fact that we do have made a lot of us have increased pounds stored up in different parts of our bodies, including the lower abdomen.

The fact that the female's metabolism rate has reduced, as well as her having reduced hormones, she may have to battle with a menopause pot belly.

There are other reasons a lot of ladies have issues shedding weight as quickly as their male counterparts, but this doesn't in any way mean that you won't do well with the keto diet.

Research has shown that embracing the keto lifestyle, as a female comes with a lot of benefits when we look at the health aspect.

When you begin keto, your body no longer runs on carbs, or use glucose as its energy source. Instead, it makes use of fat, especially those stored up fats in your body.

Weight Loss Tips

Keep Your Carbs Very Low

This is the most significant thing while on keto. Maintaining your carbs low helps to get the body into ketosis.

Do not cheat as that will hinder your success and slow the process of your body adapting to ketosis. I once tried cheating during the early stages of my keto journey but then swore never to do it again. "I had made the decision myself, and therefore when I cheat, I am only doing to myself," I told myself. Therefore, I advise you to never cheat during your keto journey.

Track Your Calories and Macros

This is very important while on the keto diet. Carbs are almost everywhere out there, and you need to keep track of all that you eat.

Watch Your Electrolytes

Electrolytes are of great essence on keto diet as they are removed from the body system.

Ensure that that you take enough potassium, magnesium, and sodium to curb excessive hunger, cramps, water retention, headaches, and cravings.

Be patient

Losing weight does not come overnight. You must consistently work hard over a long period of time in order to achieve this goal. Keto diet is a great diet if you want to lose weight. However, you need to know that the weight cannot be lost in a fortnight.

Enough Sleep and Rest

Stress levels in a person are also a factor in losing weight. When you are more stressed, the level of cortisol increases, which in turn causes weight gain or retention.

Rest is also another factor that is very important. Most people require seven to nine hours of sleep for proper rest of the body each night.

If you are enjoying and finding this book helpful, kindly leave a short review on Amazon, it means a lot to me! Thank you.

Chapter 7: 30-Day Meal Plan

1500Kcal

The values of macronutrients (carbs, protein and fats) are expressed in grams.

DAY	1	2	3	4	5
Breakfast	Avo-Tacos	Asian Chickpea Pancake	Tiramisu Chia Pudding	Vegan Breakfast Hash	Southwestern Breakfast
Lunch	Truffle Parmesan Salad	Cashew Siam Salad	Cauliflower Sushi	Flourless Bread	Spinach and Mashed Tofu Salad
Snack	Vegan Papaya Mousse	Avocado Mint Ice Cream	Vegetable Latkes	Chocolate nuts Pralines	Chocolate Peanut Butter Cookies
Dinner	Stuffed Zucchini	Fatty Choco Bombs	Shirataki noodles	Veggie Protein Bowl	Zucchini noodles Alfredo
Tot Carbs	39	49	29	29	26
Tot Prot	28	49	37	34	41
Tot Fat	104	48	55	57	53
Tot Kcal	1011	1249	2361	754	1428

12	11	10	9	8	7	6
Asian Chickpea Pancake	Southwestern Breakfast	Vegan Breakfast Muffins	Quick Breakfast Yogurt	Avo-Tacos	Tiramisu Chia Pudding	Meat-Free Breakfast Chili
Cashew Siam Salad	Hazelnut honey bread	Spinach and Mashed Tofu Salad	Mozzarella noodles	Cauliflower Sushi	Hazelnut honey bread	Walnut & Mushroom Loaf
Coconut Chia Macarons	Chocolate nuts Pralines	Vegan Cheese Fondue	Vegetable Latkes	Chocolate nuts Pralines	Avocado Mint Ice Cream	Vegan Cheese Fondue
Fatty Choco Bombs	Palmini noodles	Zucchini noodles Alfredo	Veggie Protein Bowl	Mozz. oregano bread	Shirataki noodles	Fatty Choco Bombs
49	37	32	23	31	23	27
20	46	29	35	20	14	30
49	30	56	79	56	43	47
1507	1172	1495	1204	1309	1483	1210

19	18	17	16	15	14	13
Southwestern Breakfast	Meat-Free Breakfast Chili	Avo-Tacos	Quick Breakfast Yogurt	Tiramisu Chia Pudding	Vegan Breakfast Hash	Meat-Free Breakfast Chili
Flourless Bread	Spinach and Mashed Tofu Salad	Hazelnut honey bread	Cauliflower Sushi	Walnut & Mushroom Loaf	Mozzarella noodles	Cauliflower Sushi
Chocolate Peanut Butter Cookies	Vegan Cheese Fondue	Chocolate Peanut Butter Cookies	Vegetable Latkes	Chocolate nuts Pralines	Avocado Mint Ice Cream	Chocolate Peanut Butter Cookies
Fatty Choco Bombs	Mozz. oregano bread	Palmini noodles	Veggie Protein Bowl	Fatty Choco Bombs	Shirataki noodles	Zucchini noodles Alfredo
38	28	28	27	25	21	26
50	43	32	30	28	39	40
52	33	59	86	50	49	55
1059	1575	1124	1394	1094	1292	1351

49

	20	21	22	23	24	25	26
	Vegan Breakfast Hash	Asian Chickpea Pancake	Meat-Free Breakfast Chili	Vegan Breakfast Muffins	Avo-Tacos	Quick Breakfast Yogurt	Vegan Breakfast Hash
	Hazelnut honey bread	Mozzarella noodles	Walnut & Mushroom Loaf	Mozzarella noodles	Cashew Siam Salad	Flourless Bread	Spinach and Mashed Tofu Salad
	Chocolate nuts Pralines	Avocado Mint Ice Cream	Chocolate Peanut Butter Cookies	Vegetable Latkes	Vegan Cheese Fondue	Coconut Chia Macarons	Chocolate nuts Pralines
	Shirataki noodles	Mozz. oregano bread	Zucchini noodles Alfredo	Palmini noodles	Veggie Protein Bowl	Mozz. oregano bread	Zucchini noodles Alfredo
	56	50	37	35	39	45	28
	35	42	39	38	48	30	35
	74	35	59	47	87	87	48
	1510	1356	1357	1169	1337	1515	1242

30	29	28	27
Tiramisu Chia Pudding	Asian Chickpea Pancake	Southwestern Breakfast	Vegan Breakfast Muffins
Walnut & Mushroom Loaf	Cauliflower Sushi	Flourless Bread	Cashew Siam Salad
Avocado Mint Ice Cream	Vegetable Latkes	Vegan Cheese Fondue	Chocolate Peanut Butter Cookies
Veggie Protein Bowl	Shirataki noodles	Palmini noodles	Fatty Choco Bombs
37	43	37	33
36	46	37	29
60	70	69	70
1124	1376	1424	1514

2000 Kcal

The values of macronutrients (carbs, protein and fats) are expressed in grams.

Day	Breakfast	Lunch	Snack	Dinner	Tot Carbs	Tot Pro	Tot Fat	Tot Kcal
1	Fat-Bomb Frappuccino	Avoc. Cauliflower Hummus	Piña Colada Cupcakes	7-minute noodles	32	54	115	1943
2	Banana Hazelnut Waffles	Savory Coconut Pancake	Avocado Lassi	Choco-Peppermint Bites	44	47	124	2058
3	Tofu Spinach Frittata	Kale pasta	Baked Jelly Doughnuts	Kelp noodles	34	64	92	1523
4	Egg Roll Bowl	Almond Bread	Moutabelle	Cumin bread	37	37	68	2034
5	Tofu Broccoli Scramble	Avoc. Cauliflwr Humus	Vegan Papaya Mousse	Avocado Fries	28	39	116	1655

6	7	8	9	10	11	12
Fat-Bomb Frappuccino	Matcha Avocado Pancakes	Banana Hazelnut Waffles	Avocado Mug Bread	Tofu Spinach Frittata	Fat-Bomb Frappuccino	Tofu Broccoli Scramble
Cheese head gnocchi	Savory Coconut Pancake	Kale pasta	Almond Bread	Avoc. Cauliflower Hummus	Cheese head gnocchi	7-minute noodles
Piña Colada Cupcakes	Avocado Lassi	Cinnamon raisin bread	Moutabelle	Baked Jelly Doughnuts	Vegan Papaya Mousse	Avocado Lassi
Choco-Peppermint Bites	7-minute noodles	Baked spaghetti squash	Kelp noodles	Avocado Fries	Choco-Peppermint Bites	Cumin bread
35	24	36	33	29	30	32
35	43	23	45	37	44	36
103	92	87	90	110	96	87
1856	1697	1618	1954	1637	1613	1736

13	14	15	16	17	18	19
Matcha Avocado Pancakes	Egg Roll Bowl	Avocado Mug Bread	Tofu Spinach Frittata	Avocado Mug Bread	Banana Hazelnut Waffles	Tofu Broccoli Scramble
Savory Coconut Pancake	Cheese head gnocchi	Kale pasta	Almond Bread	Avoc. Cauliflower Humus	Savory Coconut Pancake	7-minute noodles
Piña Colada Cupcakes	Cinnamon raisin bread	Moutabelle	Baked Jelly Doughnuts	Piña Colada Cupcakes	Avocado Lassi	Cinnamon raisin bread
Kelp noodles	7-minute noodles	Avocado Fries	Baked spaghetti squash	Choco-Peppermint Bites	Cumin bread	Baked spaghetti squash
35	40	36	35	32	28	30
45	36	42	36	36	36	43
78	89	80	83	87	101	87
1751	1675	1764	1503	2006	1670	1723

20	21	22	23	24	25	26
Fat-Bomb Frappuccino	Avocado Mug Bread	Egg Roll Bowl	Banana Hazelnut Waffles	Matcha Avocado Pancakes	Tofu Spinach Frittata	Tofu Broccoli Scramble
Kale pasta	Cheese head gnocchi	Almond Bread	Savory Coconut Pancake	Avoc. Cauliflower Hummus	7-minute noodles	Cheese head gnocchi
Moutabelle	Vegan Papaya Mousse	Avocado Lassi	Baked Jelly Doughnuts	Cinnamon raisin bread	Piña Colada Cupcakes	Vegan Papaya Mousse
Kelp noodles	Avocado Fries	Cumin bread	Choco-Peppermint Bites	Baked spaghetti squash	Cumin bread	Baked spaghetti squash
33	32	21	25	26	25	33
24	32	43	35	45	43	39
88	79	91	78	84	80	101
1685	1730	1964	1804	1855	1633	1751

55

27	28	29	30
Egg Roll Bowl	Banana Hazelnut Waffles	Fat-Bomb Frappuccino	Tofu Spinach Frittata
Kale pasta	Almond Bread	Avoc. Cauliflower Hummus	Savory Coconut Pancake
Moutabelle	Avocado Lassi	Baked Jelly Doughnuts	Piña Colada Cupcakes
Avocado Fries	Kelp noodles	7-minute noodles	Choco-Peppermint Bites
30	32	34	35
40	32	43	35
74	78	88	75
1566	1587	1677	1977

2500 Kcal

The values of macronutrients (carbs, protein and fats) are expressed in grams.

DAY	1	2	3	4	5
Breakfast	Keto Porridge	Spiced Breakfast Smoothie	Fat-Bomb Frappuccino	Tofu Broccoli Scramble	Overnight Oat Bowl
Lunch	Zoodles Avocado	Chicken Breast Zucchini Salad	Zoodles Avocado	Almond Bread	Curried Pumpkin Soup
Snack	Moutabelle	Cucumber Edamame Salad	Coconut Chia Macarons	Bulgogi-Spiced Tofu Wraps	Avocado Mint Ice Cream
Dinner	Rosemary bread	Soy flour noodles	Cashew Cocoa Bombs	Chicken Breast Zucchini Salad	Veggie Protein Bowl
Tot Carbs	28	37	23	37	40
Tot Pro	20	42	21	70	70
Tot Fat:	70	118	110	86	88
Tot Kcal	2202	2110	2489	2331	2343

12	11	10	9	8	7	6
Banana Hazelnut Waffles	Overnight Oat Bowl	Fat-Bomb Frappuccino	Tofu Broccoli Scramble	Banana Hazelnut Waffles	Keto Porridge	Spiced Breakfast Smoothie
Zoodles Avocado	Almond Bread	Chicken Breast Zucchini Salad	Cucumber Edamame Salad	Zoodles Avocado	Soy flour noodles	Chicken Breast Zucchini Salad
Bulgogi-Spiced Tofu Wraps	Moutabelle	Cashew Cocoa Bombs	Bulgogi-Spiced Tofu Wraps	Avocado Mint Ice Cream	Coconut Chia Macarons	Curried Pumpkin Soup
Onion black pepper bread	Rosemary bread	Veggie Protein Bowl	Chicken Breast Zucchini Salad	Rosemary bread	Veggie Protein Bowl	Cashew Cocoa Bombs
34	36	36	48	35	25	44
44	75	56	48	53	45	76
74	101	78	99	78	66	112
2093	2165	2463	2344	2447	2149	2536

13	14	15	16	17	18	19
Matcha Avocado Pancakes	Avocado Mug Bread	Keto Porridge	Spiced Breakfast Smoothie	Fat-Bomb Frappuccino	Tofu Broccoli Scramble	Overnight Oat Bowl
Curried Pumpkin Soup	Cucumber Edamame Salad	Almond Bread	Chicken Breast Zucchini Salad	Zoodles Avocado	Curried Pumpkin Soup	Soy flour noodles
Coconut Chia Macarons	Avocado Mint Ice Cream	Chicken Breast Zucchini Salad	Bulgogi-Spiced Tofu Wraps	Coconut Chia Macarons	Bulgogi-Spiced Tofu Wraps	Mouttabelle
Chicken Breast Zucchini Salad	Cashew Cocoa Bombs	Avocado Mint Ice Cream	Rosemary bread	Onion black pepper bread	Chicken Breast Zucchini Salad	Onion black pepper bread
46	41	36	33	45	49	29
65	68	56	45	53	60	58
80	90	74	86	99	76	71
2316	2254	2419	2201	2143	2444	2003

20	21	22	23	24	25	26
Banana Hazelnut Waffles	Avocado Mug Bread	Matcha Avocado Pancakes	Spiced Breakfast Smoothie	Keto Porridge	Banana Hazelnut Waffles	Tofu Broccoli Scramble
Zoodles Avocado	Cucumber Edamame Salad	Curried Pumpkin Soup	Zoodles Avocado	Chicken Breast Zucchini Salad	Almond Bread	Zoodles Avocado
Avocado Mint Ice Cream	Bulgogi-Spiced Tofu Wraps	Coconut Chia Macarons	Cucumber Edamame Salad	Onion black pepper bread	Cashew Cocoa Bombs	Cucumber Edamame Salad
Veggie Protein Bowl	Cashew Cocoa Bombs	Chicken Breast Zucchini Salad	Rosemary bread	Soy flour noodles	Veggie Protein Bowl	Chicken Breast Zucchini Salad
46	38	44	39	47	40	33
65	34	53	66	44	32	40
111	85	70	72	98	102	80
2146	2308	2193	2301	2404	2190	2318

30	29	28	27
Keto Porridge	Spiced Breakfast Smoothie	Overnight Oat Bowl	Fat-Bomb Frappuccino
Almond Bread	Zoodles Avocado	Cucumber Edamame Salad	Chicken Breast Zucchini Salad
Onion black pepper bread	Moutabelle	Cashew Cocoa Bombs	Curried Pumpkin Soup
Rosemary bread	Cashew Cocoa Bombs	Veggie Protein Bowl	Soy flour noodles
47	48	45	26
42	43	32	28
93	91	70	83
2476	2268	2486	2485

The complete list of recipes is as follows, for the page number, refer to the initial index.

7-minute noodles

Almond-Chia Doughnut Holes

Avocado and Cauliflower Hummus

Avocado Chocolate Pudding

Avocado Fries

Avocado Lassi

Avocado Mug Bread

Avocado Spring Rolls

Avo-Tacos

Baked spaghetti squash (with meatballs and marinara)

Banana Hazelnut Waffles

Beef Filled Lettuce Wraps

Berry Acai Breakfast Smoothie

Bread with Beef

Bulgogi-Spiced Tofu Wraps

Butternut squash noodles.

Cashew Cocoa Bombs

Cashew Siam Salad

Cauliflower Curry Soup

Cauliflower Sushi

Cheese head gnocchi

Cheese sausage bread

Cheesecake Cups

Chicken Breast & Zucchini Salad

Chocolate Macadamia Pralines

Chocolate Peanut Butter Cookies

Cinnamon raisin bread

Cinnamon-Vanilla Bites

Coconut Crepes

Coconut milk bread

Crispy Tofu Burgers

Cucumber Edamame Salad

Cumin bread

Curried Pumpkin Soup

Curry-Spiked Vegetable Latkes

Dairy-Free Avocado and Mint Ice Cream

Egg Roll Bowl

Fat-Bomb Frappuccino

Fatty Chocolate Bombs

Fettuccine

Flourless Bread

Garlic bread

Gingerbread-Spiced Breakfast Smoothie

Hazelnut honey bread

Italian olive herb bread

Italian raisin rosemary bread

Kale pasta

Kelp noodle salad.

Kelp noodles (with sesame chicken)

Keto Breakfast Porridge

Keto Choco "Oats"

Keto Curry Almond Bread

Lemon Rosemary Almond Slices

Low carb fettuccine Alfredo

Low-Carb Breakfast "Couscous"

Matcha Avocado Pancakes

Meat spaghetti

Meat-Free Breakfast Chili

Moutabelle with Keto Flatbread

Mozzarella noodles

Mozzarella oregano bread

Mushroom Zoodle Pasta

No-Bake Coconut Chia Macaroons

Onion black pepper bread

Overnight Oat Bowl

Palmini noodles (with sausage ragu)

Peanut Butter Bombs

Piña Colada Cupcakes

Quick Breakfast Yogurt

Quick Veggie Protein Bowl

Raw Zoodles with Avocado 'N Nuts

Sausage bread

Savory Coconut Pancake

Shirataki noodles (with mushrooms)

Soy flour noodles   106

Spiced Tofu and Broccoli Scramble

Spicy Satay Tofu Salad 120

Spinach and Mashed Tofu Salad

Stove made Keto Cauliflower Mac and cheese.

Stuffed Zucchini

Sugar and Cinnamon Mug cake

Tangy Green Salad

The Asian Chickpea Pancake

Tiramisu Chia Pudding

Tofu and Spinach Frittata

Tofu Cheese Nuggets & Zucchini Fries

Truffle Parmesan Salad

Vegan Baked Jelly Doughnuts

Vegan Banana Bread

Vegan Breakfast Biscuits

Vegan Breakfast Hash

Vegan Breakfast Muffins

Vegan Breakfast Sausages

Vegan Breakfast Skillet

Vegan Cheese Fondue 217

Vegan Choco-Peppermint Bites

Vegan Crème Brulee

Vegan Fudge Revel BarsVegan Papaya Mousse

Vegan Southwestern Breakfast

Vizza

Walnut & Mushroom Loaf

Zoodle Pesto Salad

Zucchini noodles Alfredo

Chapter 8: Breakfast Recipes

Avo-Tacos

Prep time: 15 minutes

Cook time: 5 minutes

Serves: 4

Ingredients

- 30 milliliters, Avocado Oil
- 60 g, Cauliflower Rice
- 58 g, Walnuts or Pecans, crushed
- 14 g, Chipotle Chili, chopped
- 14 g, Jalapeno Pepper, minced
- 20 g Onions, chopped
- 2.5 g Cumin
- 2.5 g salt, sea salt preferred
- 100 g, Tomato, ripe, diced
- 2 tablespoons, Lime Juice

Instructions:

1. The Avo-Taco is so easy to make that you'll want to do this every week. Start by grabbing a bowl and putting the salsa ingredients together; in a small bowl, you'll need the diced tomatoes, jalapeno, the onion, and half of the lime. If you want, you can add in a bit of cilantro to give it a bit more freshness, and don't forget to add the salt!

2. Once you're done, put a frying pan on medium heat and add the avocado oil and let it heat. In the meantime, you can get together the rest of the ingredients, including the cauliflower-rice (which you can totally make at home if you want--it's a 5-minute blend job), and toss in everything but the avocado, and cook on low to medium heat for about 5 minutes. Add the mixture to the avocado halves and top with salsa and munch away!

Nutritional Value Per Serving:

Calories 179

Carbohydrates 13 g

Fats 28.24 g

Protein 4 g

The Asian Chickpea Pancake

Prep time: 5 minutes

Cook time: 10 minutes

Serves: 1

Ingredients:

- 34 grams Green Onion, chopped
- 34 grams Red Pepper, thinly sliced
- 70 grams Chickpea Powder
- 1.5 grams, Garlic Powder
- 1.25 grams, Baking Powder
- 1 .5 grams, Salt
- 0.25 gram, Chili Flakes

Instructions

1. This chickpea pancake is super easy. Take your vegetables, prep them, then mix everything else, starting from the chickpea flour to the chili flakes in a bowl. Whisk until you see air bubbles, just like you would for a normal pancake.

2. Add the chopped veggies and after one final stir, add the mixture to a preheated skillet and allow it to spread evenly over the pan for about 5 minutes. Once the underside is cooked through, flip and let it cook for an additional 5 minutes, and once you are done, simply plate and serve.

Nutritional Value Per Serving:

Calories 227

Carbohydrates 38 g

Fats 3.6 g

Protein 12 g

Overnight Oat Bowl

Prep time: 10 minutes

Cook time: 10 minutes

Serves: 2

Ingredients

- 15 grams, Chia Seeds
- 75 grams, Hemp Hearts
- 14 grams, Sweetener
- 2/3 Cup, Coconut Milk
- ¼ grams, Vanilla Extract/Vanilla Bean
- 1.25 grams of Salt

Instructions

1. Thoroughly mix in all of your ingredients and allow the bowl to sit overnight in a covered container to avoid evaporation. You want the oats to sit for at least 8 hours, so if you have a long night ahead of you, plan accordingly.

Nutritional Value Per Serving

Calories 634

Carbohydrates 17 g

Fats 52.32 g

Protein 27.75 g

Coconut Crepes

Prep time: 10 minutes

Cook time: 8 minutes

Serves: 3

Ingredients

- 15 grams Virgin Coconut Oil
- ¼ cup, Almond Milk
- ¼ cup, Coconut Milk
- ¼ grams, Vanilla Essence
- 30 grams, Coconut Flour
- 15 grams, Almond Meal
- 1 cup Applesauce

Instructions

2. Coconut crepes, in addition to being super delicious, also happen to be very easy to whip up. Dump all of your ingredients into one large bowl and whisk until smooth. Then set aside for ten minutes to allow the liquid to absorb into the flour. In the meantime, lightly oil a frying pan on the stove, and pour in the batter and spread until the pan is coated with a thin layer.

3. Cook until the crepe starts to get crispy, and flip. Another minute on the stove, and you are ready to serve alongside your toppings of choice or course.

Nutritional Value Per Serving

Calories 437

Carbohydrates 12.15 g

Fats 16.54 g

Protein 1 g

Matcha Avocado Pancakes

Prep time: 10 minutes

Cook time: 5 minutes

Serves: 6

Ingredients:

- 1 cup Almond Flour
- 1 medium-sized avocado, mashed
- 1 cup Coconut Milk
- 1 tbsp Matcha Powder
- ½ tsp Baking Soda
- ¼ tsp Salt

Instructions:

1. Mix all ingredients into a batter.
2. To thin the mixture out, add water as need be.
3. Lightly oil a non-stick pan.
4. Scoop about a third cup of the batter and cook over medium heat until bubbly on the surface(about 2-3 minutes).
5. Cook for 1 minute on the other side.

Nutritional Value Per Serving:

Calories 179

Carbohydrates 5 g

Fats 14 g

Protein 1 g

Low-Carb Breakfast "Couscous"

Prep time: 10 minutes

Cook time: 2 minutes

Serves: 4

Ingredients:

- 200 grams Cauliflower, riced
- 30 g Strawberries
- 20 g Almonds
- 20 g Flax Seeds
- 60 g Mandarin Segments
- 1 cup Coconut Milk
- 1 tbsp. Erythritol
- ¼ tsp. Cinnamon Powder
- 3 tbsp. Rose Water

Instructions:

1. Mix all ingredients in a bowl (microwave safe)).
2. Cook for 2 minutes at 30-second intervals.

Nutritional Value Per Serving:

Calories 490

Carbohydrates 9 g

Fats 17 g

Protein 3 g

Gingerbread-Spiced Breakfast Smoothie

Prep time: 2 minutes

Cook time: 0 minutes

Serves: 2

Ingredients:

- 1 cup Coconut Milk
- 1 bag Tea
- ¼ tsp Cinnamon Powder
- 1/8 tsp Nutmeg Powder
- 1/8 tsp Powdered Cloves
- 1/3 cup Chia Seeds
- 2 tbsp Flax Seeds

Instructions:

1. Place the teabag in a cup and pour in hot water. Allow to steep for a few minutes.
2. Pour the tea into a blender together with the rest of the ingredients. Process until smooth.

Nutritional Value Per Serving:

Calories 649

Carbohydrates 10 g

Fats 46 g

Protein 6 g

Vegan Breakfast Muffins

Prep time: 5 minutes

Cook time: 3 minutes

Serves: 3

Ingredients:
- 2 tbsp Almond Flour
- ½ tsp Baking Powder
- ½ tsp Salt
- 2 tbsp Ground Flax Seeds
- ¼ cup Coconut Milk
- 3 tbsp Avocado Oil

Instructions:
1. Whisk together almond flour, ground flax, baking powder, and salt in a bowl.
2. Stir in coconut milk
3. Heat avocado oil in a non-stick pan.
4. Ladle in the batter and cook for 2-3 minutes per side.

Nutritional Value Per Serving:

Calories 194

Carbohydrates 2 g

Fats 21 g

Protein 1 g

Vegan Breakfast Biscuits

Prep time: 10 minutes

Cook time: 10 minutes

Serves: 6

Ingredients:

- 1.5 cups Almond Flour
- 1 tbsp Baking Powder
- ¼ tsp Salt
- ½ tsp Onion Powder
- ½ cup Coconut Milk
- ¼ cup Nutritional Yeast
- 2 tbsp Ground Flax Seeds
- ¼ cup Olive Oil

Instructions:

1. Preheat oven to 450°F.
2. Whisk together all ingredients in a bowl.
3. Divide the batter into a pre-greased muffin tin.
4. Bake for 10 minutes.

Nutritional Value Per Serving:

Calories 406

Carbohydrates 10 g

Fats 28 g

Protein 7 g

Avocado Mug Bread

Prep time: 2 minutes

Cook time: 2 minutes

Serves: 1

Ingredients:

- ¼ cup Almond Flour
- ½ tsp Baking Powder
- ¼ tsp Salt
- ¼ cup Mashed Avocados
- 1 tbsp Coconut Oil

Instructions:

1. Mix all ingredients in a microwave-safe mug.
2. Microwave for 90 seconds.
3. Cool for 2 minutes.

Nutritional Value Per Serving:

Calories 317

Carbohydrates 9 g

Fats 30 g

Protein 6 g

Vegan Breakfast Sausages

Prep time: 15 minutes

Cook time: 12 minutes

Serves: 4

Ingredients:

- 200 grams Portobella Mushrooms
- 150 grams Walnuts
- 1 tbsp Tomato Paste
- 75 grams Panko
- 1 tsp Paprika
- 1 tsp Dried Sage
- 1 tsp Salt
- ½ tsp Black Pepper

Instructions:

1. Blend all ingredients in a food processor.
2. Divide mixture into serving-sized portions and shape into sausages.
3. Bake for 12 minutes at 375°F.
4. Serve.

Nutritional Value Per Serving:

Calories 371

Carbohydrates 9 g

Fats 25 g

Protein 7 g

Quick Breakfast Yogurt

Prep time: 2 minutes

Cook time: 8 minutes

Serves: 6

Ingredients:

- 4 cups Full-Fat Coconut Milk
- 2 tbsp Coconut Milk Powder
- 100 grams Strawberries, for serving

Instructions:

1. Whisk together coconut milk and milk powder in a microwave-safe bowl.
2. Heat on high for 8-9 minutes.
3. Top with fresh strawberries and choice of sweetener to serve.

Nutritional Value Per Serving:

Calories 186

Carbohydrates 10 g

Fats 38 g

Protein 4 g

Spiced Tofu and Broccoli Scramble

Prep time: 5 minutes

Cook time: 3 minutes

Serves: 3

Ingredients:

- 400 grams Firm Tofu, drained and pressed
- 1 tbsp Tamari
- 1 tbsp Garlic Powder
- 2 tsp Paprika Powder
- 2 tsp Turmeric Powder
- 150 grams Broccoli, rough-chopped
- 2 tbsp Olive Oil

Instructions:

1. Crumble the tofu in a bowl with the garlic powder, paprika, turmeric, and nutritional yeast.
2. Heat olive oil in a pan.
3. Sautee broccoli for a minute.
4. Stir in spiced tofu. Cook for 1-2 minutes.
5. Season with tamari.
6. Serve hot.

Nutritional Value Per Serving:

Calories 331

Carbohydrates 7 g

Fats 17 g

Protein 16 g

Meat-Free Breakfast Chili

Prep time: 10 minutes

Cook time: 20 minutes

Serves: 4

Ingredients:

- 400 grams Textured-Vegetable Protein
- ¼ cup Red Kidney Beans
- ½ cup Canned Diced Tomatoes
- 1 Large Bell Pepper, diced
- 1 Large White Onion, diced
- 1 tsp Cumin Powder
- 1 tsp Chili Powder
- 1 tsp Paprika
- 1 tsp Garlic Powder
- ½ tsp Dried Oregano
- 2 cups Water

Instructions:

1. Combine all ingredients in a pot.
2. Simmer for 20 minutes.
3. Serve with your favorite bread or some slices of fresh avocado.

Nutritional Value Per Serving:

Calories 174

Carbohydrates 9 g

Fats 9 g

Protein 18 g

Vegan Southwestern Breakfast

Prep time: 10 minutes

Cook time: 5 minutes

Serves: 6

Ingredients:

- 1 small White Onion, diced
- 1 Bell Pepper, diced
- 150 grams Mushrooms, sliced
- 400 grams Firm Tofu, crumbled
- 1 tsp Turmeric Powder
- 1 tbsp Garlic Powder
- 2 tbsp Nutritional Yeast
- ¼ cup Chopped Green Onions
- 2 cups Fresh Spinach
- 1 cup Cherry Tomatoes
- 2 cups Baked Beans
- 2 tbsp Olive Oil

Instructions:

1. Sautee onions, bell peppers, and mushrooms until onions are translucent.
2. Add in the tofu.
3. Stir in the turmeric, garlic powder, and nutritional yeast.

4. Add green onions and spinach. Sautee for 1-2 minutes.

5. Serve with baked beans and cherry tomatoes.

Nutritional Value Per Serving:

Calories 174

Carbohydrates 10 g

Fats 10 g

Protein 13 g

Egg Roll Bowl

Prep time: 5 minutes

Cook time: 6 minutes

Serves: 2

Ingredients:

- 2 7-oz. packs shirataki noodles
- 1 tbsp. coconut oil
- 1 tbsp. sesame oil
- 1 tbsp. rice vinegar
- 1 12-oz. pack extra firm tofu, drained, cubed
- 1 red onion, diced
- 2 garlic cloves, minced
- 1-inch fresh ginger, finely minced
- 4 tbsp. low sodium soy sauce
- ½ cup red pickled cabbage, chopped
- ½ cup carrots, matchsticks or julienned

Instructions:

1. In a medium bowl, rinse the shirataki noodles with cold water, drain, and set aside.
2. Put a large skillet over medium-high heat.
3. Add the coconut oil and sesame oil to the skillet.
4. Add the rice vinegar, tofu cubes, and onions to the skillet. Stir-fry the ingredients until the onions start to caramelize.

5. Blend in the garlic, ginger, and soy sauce. Cook for a minute while occasionally stirring.
6. Add carrots and cook for 5 more minutes while stirring occasionally.
7. Take the skillet off the heat, divide the shirataki noodles over 2 medium bowls, top each portion with half of the tofu mixture and chopped cabbage, serve, and enjoy!

Nutritional Value Per Serving:

Calories 319

Carbohydrates 10 g

Fats 17.6 g

Protein 16.7 g

Keto Breakfast Porridge

Prep time: 5 minutes

Cook time: 5 minutes

Serves: 4

Ingredients:

- 1 cup Flaked Coconut
- ½ cup Hemp Seeds
- 1 tbsp Coconut Flour
- 1 cup Water
- ½ cup Coconut Cream
- 1 tbsp Ground Cinnamon
- 1 tbsp Erythritol

Instructions:

1. Combine all ingredients in a pot.
2. Simmer for 5 minutes, stirring continuously.

Nutritional Value Per Serving:

Calories 402

Carbohydrates 9 g

Fats 18 g

Protein 4 g

Berry Acai Breakfast Smoothie

Prep time: 2 minutes

Serves: 1

Ingredients:

- 1 cup Silk Tofu
- 2 tbsp Coconut Cream
- 1 cup Ice Cubes
- ¼ cup Raspberries
- 2 tbsp Acai Powder
- 3 tbsp Soy Protein Powder

Instructions:

1. Combine all ingredients in a blender.
2. Blend until smooth.

Nutritional Value Per Serving:

Calories 556

Carbohydrates 10 g

Fats 20 g

Protein 18 g

Keto Choco "Oats"

Prep time: 5 minutes

Cook time: 5 minutes

Serves: 2

Ingredients:

- 200 grams Cauliflower, riced
- 1 cup Coconut Milk
- 2 tbsp Flax Seeds
- 1 tbsp Erythritol
- 2 tbsp Cocoa Powder
- 1 tbsp Vanilla Extract
- 50 grams fresh Raspberries
- 1 tbsp Cacao Nibs

Instructions:

1. Combine cauliflower, coconut milk, flax seeds, erythritol, cocoa powder, and vanilla extract in a pot.
2. Simmer for 3-5 minutes.
3. Ladle into bowls and top with fresh raspberries and cacao nibs.

Nutritional Value Per Serving:

Calories 564

Carbohydrates 10 g

Fats 41 g

Protein 22 g

Banana Hazelnut Waffles

Prep time: 3 minutes

Cook time: 5 minutes

Serves: 2

Ingredients:

- 2 tbsp Flaxseed Meal
- 1/2 cup Almond Flour
- 2 tbsp Erythritol
- 1 tsp Baking Powder
- 1 tsp Ground Cinnamon
- 2 tbsp Hazelnut Butter
- ½ cup Coconut Milk
- 1 tsp Banana Essence

Instructions:

1. Blend the ingredients until smooth.
2. Pour into waffle iron and cook for 3-5 minutes.

Nutritional Value Per Serving:

Calories 316

Carbohydrates 9 g

Fats 31 g

Protein 3 g

Vegan Breakfast Skillet

Prep time: 3 minutes

Cook time: 5 minutes

Serves: 4

Ingredients:

- 3 tbsp Olive Oil
- 400 g Firm Tofu, drained and crumbled
- 20 g Chickpeas
- 100 g Spinach
- 1 tbsp g Powder
- 1 tsp Paprika
- ½ tsp Turmeric Powder
- ¼ tsp Salt
- ¼ tsp Pepper

Instructions:

1. Heat olive oil in a skillet.
2. Add tofu and stir for about 3 minutes.
3. Stir in all the spices.
4. Add chickpeas and spinach. Saute for another minute.
5. Serve hot.

Nutritional Value Per Serving:

Calories 271

Carbohydrates   10 g

Fats 19 g

Protein 18 g

Vegan Breakfast Hash

Prep time: 15 minutes

Cook time: 5 minutes

Serves: 4

Ingredients:

- 1 cup Cooked Quinoa
- 1 cup Shredded Broccoli
- 2 tbsp Flax Seed
- ½ cup Coconut Flour
- 1 tsp Garlic Powder
- 1 tsp Onion Powder
- 2 tbsp Coconut Oil

Instructions:

1. Stir flax seeds with half a cup of water in a large mixing bowl. Leave for a few minutes.
2. Stir in all remaining ingredients.
3. Form the mixture into patties.
4. Heat vegetable oil in a pan.
5. Fry each side of the patties for 2-3 minutes.

Nutritional Value Per Serving:

Calories 135

Carbohydrates 10 g

Fats 10 g

Protein 3 g

Tiramisu Chia Pudding

Prep time: 15 minutes

Cook time: 5 minutes

Serves: 1

Ingredients:

- ¼ cup Chia Seeds
- 2 tsp Instant Coffee
- 2 tbsp Coconut Cream
- ¾ cup Water
- 1 tbsp Erythritol
- 1 tsp Powdered Cinnamon

Instructions:

1. Combine all ingredients in a mason jar.
2. Shake until well blended.
3. Chill for at least 20 minutes.

Nutritional Value Per Serving:

Calories 112

Carbohydrates 9 g

Fats 9 g

Protein 3 g

Tofu and Spinach Frittata

Prep time: 15 minutes

Cook time: 5 minutes

Serves: 4

Ingredients:

- 400 grams Firm Tofu
- 2 tbsp tamari
- 2 tbsp Nutritional Yeast
- 1 tsp Turmeric
- 1 tbsp Garlic Powder
- 2 cups Baby Spinach, chopped
- 1 Red Bell Pepper, chopped
- 2 tbsp Olive Oil

Instructions:

1. Combine tofu, tamari, nutritional yeast, turmeric, and garlic powder in a food processor. Blend until smooth.
2. Fold in the spinach and bell pepper into the mixture.
3. Brush an iron skillet with olive oil.
4. Pour the mixture into the skillet.
5. Bake for 25 minutes at 360F.

Nutritional Value Per Serving:

Calories 236

Carbohydrates 9 g

Fats 16 g   Protein 18 g

Fat-Bomb Frappuccino

Prep time: 15 minutes

Serves: 1

Ingredients:

- 2/3 cup Brewed Coffee
- ¼ cup Almond Milk
- 2 tbsp Erythritol
- 1 tsp Vanilla Extract
- 2 tbsp Coconut Oil
- ½ cup Ice Cubes

Instructions:

1. Blend coffee, coconut oil, vanilla extract, and erythritol until smooth.

Nutritional Value Per Serving:

Calories 278

Carbohydrates 6 g

Fats 28 g

Protein 1 g

Chapter 9: Lunch Recipes

<u>Truffle Parmesan Salad</u>

Prep time: 15 minutes

Cook time: 0 minutes

Serves: 4

Ingredients:

- 4 cups kale, chopped
- ½ cup truffle parmesan cheese
- 1 tsp. Dijon mustard
- 2 tbsp. olive oil
- 2 tbsp. lemon juice
- Salt and pepper to taste
- 2 tbsp. water

Instructions:

1. Rinse the kale with cold water, then drain the kale and put it into a large bowl.
2. In a medium-sized bowl, mix the rest ingredients into a dressing.
3. Pour the dressing over the kale and stir gently to cover the kale evenly.
4. Transfer the large bowl to the fridge and allow the salad to chill for up to one hour – doing so will

guarantee a better flavor. Alternatively, the salad can be served right away. Enjoy!

Nutritional Value Per Serving:

Calories 199

Carbohydrates 10 g

Fats 16.6 g

Protein 3.5 g

Cashew Siam Salad

Prep time: 12 minutes

Cook time: 3 minutes

Serves: 4

Ingredients:
Salad:

- 4 cups baby spinach, rinsed, drained
- ½ cup pickled red cabbage

Dressing:

- 1-inch piece ginger, finely chopped
- 1 tsp. chili garlic paste
- 1 tbsp. soy sauce
- ½ tbsp. rice vinegar
- 1 tbsp. sesame oil
- 3 tbsp. avocado oil

Toppings:

- ½ cup raw cashews, unsalted
- ¼ cup fresh cilantro, chopped

Instructions:

1. Put the spinach and red cabbage in a large bowl. Toss to combine and set the salad aside.

2. Toast the cashews in a frying pan, occasionally stirring until the cashews are golden brown. This should take about 3 minutes. Turn off the heat and set the frying pan aside.

3. Mix all the dressing ingredients in a medium-sized bowl and use a spoon to mix them into a smooth dressing.

4. Pour the dressing on salad and top with the toasted cashews.

5. Toss the salad to combine all ingredients and transfer the large bowl to the fridge. Allow up to one hour to chill the salad– doing so will guarantee a better flavor. Alternatively, the salad can be served right away, topped with the optional cilantro. Enjoy!

Nutritional Value Per Serving:

Calories 236
Carbohydrates 4 g
Fats 21.6 g
Protein 4.2 g

Avocado and Cauliflower Hummus

Prep time: 5 minutes

Cook time: 20 minutes

Serves: 2

Ingredients:

- 1 medium cauliflower, stem removed and chopped
- 1 large Hass avocado, peeled, pitted, and chopped
- ¼ cup extra virgin olive oil
- 2 garlic cloves
- ½ tbsp. lemon juice
- ½ tsp. onion powder
- ¼ tsp. Sea salt
- ¼ tsp. ground black pepper
- 2 large carrots
- ¼ cup fresh cilantro, chopped

Instructions:

1. Preheat oven to 450°F, and use aluminum foil to line on a baking tray.
2. Put the chopped cauliflower on the baking tray and drizzle with 2 tablespoons of olive oil.
3. Roast the chopped cauliflower in the oven for 20-25 minutes, until lightly brown.
4. Remove the tray from the oven and allow the cauliflower to cool down.

5. Add all the ingredients—except the carrots and optional fresh cilantro—to a food processor or blender, and blend the ingredients into a smooth hummus.

6. Transfer the hummus to a medium-sized bowl, cover, and put it in the fridge for at least 30 minutes.

7. Remove the hummus from the fridge and, if desired, top it with the optional chopped cilantro and more salt and pepper to taste; serve with the carrot fries, and enjoy!

Nutritional Value Per Serving:

Calories 416

Carbohydrates 7 g

Fats 40.3 g

Protein 3.3 g

Raw Zoodles with Avocado 'N Nuts

Prep time: 10 minutes

Cook time: 0 minutes

Serves: 2

Ingredients:

- 1 medium zucchini
- 1½ cups basil
- ⅓ cup water
- 5 tbsp. pine nuts
- 2 tbsp. lemon juice
- 1 medium avocado, peeled, pitted, and sliced
- 2 tbsp. olive oil
- 6 yellow cherry tomatoes, halved
- 6 red cherry tomatoes, halved
- Sea salt and black pepper to taste

Instructions:

1. Add the basil, water, nuts, lemon juice, avocado slices, optional olive oil (if desired), salt, and pepper to a blender.

2. Blend the ingredients into a smooth mixture. Add pepper and salt to taste and blend again.

3. Divide the sauce and the zucchini noodles between two medium-sized bowls for serving, and combine in each.

4. Top the mixtures with the halved yellow cherry tomatoes, and the optional red cherry tomatoes (if desired); serve and enjoy!

Nutritional Value Per Serving:

Calories 517

Carbohydrates 5 g

Fats 28.1 g

Protein 7.2 g

Cauliflower Sushi

Prep time: 30 minutes

Cook time: 0 minutes

Serves: 4

Ingredients:
Sushi Base:

- 6 cups cauliflower florets
- ½ cup vegan cheese
- 1 medium spring onion, diced
- 4 nori sheets
- Sea salt and pepper to taste
- 1 tbsp. rice vinegar or sushi vinegar
- 1 medium garlic clove, minced

Filling:

- 1 medium Hass avocado, peeled, sliced
- ½ medium cucumber, skinned, sliced
- 4 asparagus spears
- a handful of enoki mushrooms

Instructions:

1. Add cauliflower florets in a blender or food processor. Pulse the florets into a rice-like substance. When using readymade cauliflower rice, add this to the blender.

2. Add the vegan cheese, spring onions, and vinegar to the food processor or blender. Top these ingredients with salt and pepper to taste, and pulse everything into a chunky mixture. Make sure not to turn the ingredients into a puree by pulsing too long.

3. Taste and season with pepper, salt, or vinegar. Add the optional minced garlic clove to the blender and pulse again for a few seconds.

4. Lay the nori sheets out and spread the cauliflower rice mixture out evenly between the sheets. Make sure to leave at least 2 inches of the top and bottom edges empty.

5. Place one or more combinations of multiple filling ingredients along the center of the spread-out rice mixture. Experiment with different ingredients per nori sheet for the best flavor.

6. Roll up each nori sheet tightly. (Using a sushi mat will make this easier.)

7. Either serve the sushi as a nori roll or slice each roll up into sushi pieces.

8. Serve right away with a small amount of wasabi, pickled ginger, and soy sauce!

Nutritional Value Per Serving:

Calories 189

Carbohydrates 6 g

Fats 14.4 g

Protein 6.1 g

Spinach and Mashed Tofu Salad

Prep time: 20 minutes

Serves: 4

Ingredients:

- 2 8-oz. blocks firm tofu, drained
- 4 cups baby spinach leaves
- 4 tbsp. cashew butter
- 1½ tbsp. soy sauce
- 1-inch piece ginger, finely chopped
- 1 tsp. red miso paste
- 2 tbsp. sesame seeds
- 1 tsp. organic orange zest
- 1 tsp. nori flakes
- 2 tbsp. water

Instructions:

1. Absorb any excess water left in the tofu using paper towels before crumbling both blocks into small pieces.
2. In a large bowl, combine the mashed tofu with the spinach leaves.
3. Mix the remaining ingredients in another small bowl and, if desired, add the optional water for a more smooth dressing.

4. Pour this dressing over the mashed tofu and spinach leaves.

5. Transfer the bowl to the fridge and allow the salad to chill for up to one hour. Doing so will guarantee a better flavor. Or, the salad can be served right away. Enjoy!

Nutritional Value Per Serving:

Calories 166

Carbohydrates 5 g

Fats 10.7 g

Protein 11.3 g

Keto Curry Almond Bread

Prep time: 10 minutes

Cook time: 15 minutes

Serves: 2

Ingredients:

- ½ cup almond flour
- ¼ cup almond milk
- ¼ cup ground flaxseed
- 2 tbsp. coconut oil
- 2 tbsp. red curry paste
- ½ tsp. salt
- ½ tsp. cane sugar
- 2 kaffir lime leaves, chopped
- 2 tsp. dried ginger, fresh, minced
- ¼ cup water
- 4 tbsp. coconut flakes

Instructions:

1. Line a baking sheet with parchment paper.
2. In a medium bowl, mix the almond milk with the sugar, salt, and ground flaxseeds. Stir well and let it sit for 10 minutes.
3. Add the flour, kaffir lime leaves, and ginger to the bowl.

4. Incorporate all ingredients using your hands or an electric mixer. Add some of the optional water to make the mixing easier.
5. Divide the dough into two and flatten these out onto the baking sheet.
6. Grease both sides of the dough with the coconut oil and apply a tablespoon of red curry paste on the top side of each flattened bread.
7. Allow the pieces of bread to rest for an hour at room temperature.
8. Preheat the oven to 400°F.
9. Bake the bread for about 15 minutes, until golden brown on top.
10. Top the bread with the optional coconut flakes.
11. Serve and enjoy!

Nutritional Value Per Serving:

Calories 372

Carbohydrates 8 g

Fats 34.7 g

Protein 8.3 g

Mozzarella noodles

Prep time: 5 minutes

Cook time:

Serves: 3

Ingredients:

- 1 cup shredded mozzarella cheese
- ½ cup hot water
- 4 sachets plain gelatin
- 1 teaspoon Italian seasoning
- 1 teaspoon garlic powder
- ¼ teaspoon pepper
- ¼ teaspoon salt

Instructions:

1. Add the water in a small saucepan and place on medium heat.
2. When the water starts simmering, add the gelatin and mix until it's fully dissolved.
3. Add the mozzarella.
4. Mix until the cheese melts.
5. Add the Italian seasoning, garlic powder, pepper, and salt.
6. Pour the mixture on a parchment paper-lined pan.
7. Spread it thin on the paper.
8. Let the thin spread sit for 30 minutes.

9. Use a pizza wheel to cut the spread into thin noodles.
10. Cook into a dish.

Nutritional Value Per Serving:

Calories 299

Carbohydrates 2.1g

Fats 8.4g

Protein 11.2g

7-minute noodles

Prep time: 2 minutes

Cook time: 5 minutes

Serves: 2

Ingredients:

- 1 oz. cream cheese
- 2 eggs
- ¼ tsp wheat gluten

Instructions:

1. Preheat the oven to 325°F.
2. Mix the cream cheese, eggs, and wheat gluten until smooth.
3. Pour the mixture on a silicone mat on top of a heavy baking pan.
4. Spread out into a rectangle.
5. Bake for 5 minutes.
6. Allow a few minutes to cool.
7. Use a pizza wheel to cut into noodles.

Nutritional Value Per Serving:

Calories 332

Carbohydrates 0.6g

Protein 2g

Fat 7.4g

Cheese head gnocchi

Prep time: 3 minutes

Cook time: 3 minutes

Serves: 3

Ingredients:

- 2 cups almond flour
- 2 cups mozzarella cheese, shredded
- ¼ cup butter
- 1 egg
- 1 egg yolk

Instructions:

1. In a microwave-safe dish, mix the cheese and butter and microwave for 2 minutes.
2. Mix and microwave for another minute.
3. Mix well until they're fully combined and let it cool slightly.
4. Add the egg, the egg yolk, and the almond flour.
5. Mix until a dough is formed.
6. Knead until the dough is semi-stretchy.
7. Roll into a log of 1 inch in diameter.
8. Cut small pieces and shape into disks.
9. Freeze the formed gnocchi in the freezer for 15 minutes.
10. Boil a pot of water and add a pinch of salt.

11. Add the frozen gnocchi and boil for 1-2 minutes until they're floating.

12. Cool for 5 minutes before adding any sauce.

Nutritional Value Per Serving:

Calories 305

Carbohydrates 6g

Fats 32g

Protein 25.8g

Fettuccine

Prep time: 5 minutes

Cook time: 4 minutes

Serves: 2

Ingredients:

- 3 tbsps. coconut flour
- 1 cup almond flour
- 2 tbsp. xanthan gum
- 1 egg
- ¼ tsp sea salt
- 2 tsp apple cider vinegar
- 3 tsp water
- 2 tbsps. butter
- ¼ cup heavy cream
- 2 cloves garlic
- 1 tbsp. parmesan cheese
- 1 tsp lemon zest
- salt and pepper

Instructions:

1. Mix the coconut flour, almond flour, xanthan gum, egg, sea salt, apple cider vinegar, and water together.
2. Form the dough into a ball.

3. Use a cling film to cover and let it rest in the fridge for about 30 minutes.
4. Using a rolling pin, flatten the dough until it is about half an inch thick.
5. Cut the dough into the shape of fettuccine using a pizza wheel.
6. Let the shaped pasta rest in the fridge for another 15 minutes.
7. Add the butter in a saucepan and let it brown. After, add the cream, garlic, lemon zest, and parmesan.
8. Add salt and pepper to taste.
9. Add past after the cheese is melted.
10. Cook until the pasta is cooked.

Nutritional Value Per Serving:

Calories 453

Carbohydrates 7g

Fats 23g

Protein 14g

Soy flour noodles

Prep time: 3 minutes

Cook time: 2 minutes

Serves: 3

Ingredients:

- 1 ½ cups soy flour
- ¾ cup gluten
- 2 tsp salt
- 2 tbsps. warm water
- 2 tsp olive oil

Instructions:

1. Add the soy flour, gluten, and salt in a mixing bowl and mix.
2. Add the remaining ingredients and form a dough ball.
3. Wrap in plastic film and rest in the fridge for half an hour to 45 minutes.
4. Remove the dough and cut into 8 pieces and process through your pasta cutter or use a rolling pin to flatten the dough on a flat surface and use a pizza wheel to cut into small noodles.
5. Bring a pot of water to boil.
6. Add a pinch of salt.

7. Cook the noodles for 2 minutes, drain the water, and your noodles are ready.

Nutritional Value Per Serving:

Calories 522

Carbohydrates 5.2g

Fats 15g

Protein 21g

Kale pasta

Prep time: 2 minutes

Cook time: 12 minutes

Serves: 4

Ingredients:

- 3 eggs
- 4 oz. cream cheese
- 1 cup raw kale
- ½ cup mozzarella

Instructions:

1. Preheat oven to 325°F.
2. Using a blender, blend the eggs, cream cheese, kale, and mozzarella into liquid.
3. Lay parchment paper on a baking tray.
4. Pour the liquid on the tray.
5. Bake for 10-12 minutes.
6. Remove the parchment paper and let it cool slightly.
7. Use a pizza wheel to cut the pasta into noodles or any other desired shape.

Nutritional Value Per Serving:

Calories 342

Carbohydrates 4.1 g

Fats 14 g

Protein 7.9 g

Meat spaghetti

Prep time: 2 minutes

Cook time: 20 seconds

Serves: 2

Ingredients:

- 3 cups diced chicken breast
- 2 eggs
- 1 tbsp. psyllium husk
- 1 tsp old bay seasoning

Instructions:

1. In a blender, mix the ingredients until everything is smooth and in a liquid state.
2. Put the mix in a piping bag.
3. Cut the piping bag's tip very close to the tip to make your spaghetti thin.
4. Boil water in a pot with some salt.
5. Pipe the noodles one by one.
6. Cook for only 20 seconds. The spaghetti noodles will rise to the top once done.
7. Drain all the water from the spaghetti before serving.

Nutritional Value Per Serving:

Calories 353

Carbohydrates 2.9 g

Fiber 0 g

Fats 6.8 g   Protein 42 g

Zoodle Pesto Salad

Prep time: 20 minutes

Serves: 2

Ingredients:

- 2 medium zucchinis
- ¼ cup extra virgin olive oil
- 1 ½ cups fresh baby spinach leaves
- ¼ cup walnuts, crushed
- 1 tsp. garlic powder
- ¼ tsp. Sea salt
- ¼ tsp. ground black pepper
- ¼ cup capers, chopped
- ½ cup of vegan cheese

Instructions:

1. Combine all the ingredients except the zoodles, capers, and optional vegan cheese in a food processor or blender. Pulse for 1-2 minutes into a smooth pesto.

2. If desired, cook zoodles or zucchini slices for up to 4 minutes in a large skillet, with boiling water and a pinch of olive oil, over medium heat. Alternatively, the zoodles or zucchini slices can be used raw.

3. Melt the optional vegan cheese on a plate in the microwave for about 40 seconds, until it is melted and spreadable.
4. Serve the raw or cooked zoodles with the pesto, garnished with the chopped capers. Top the dish with the optional molten vegan cheese and add more salt and pepper to taste.
5. Serve and enjoy!

Nutritional Value Per Serving:

Calories 389

Carbohydrates 3 g

Fats 37 g

Protein 5.9 g

Cucumber Edamame Salad

Prep time: 5 minutes

Cook time: 8 minutes

Serves: 2

Ingredients:

- 3 tbsp. avocado oil
- 1 cup cucumber
- ½ cup fresh sugar snap peas
- ½ cup fresh edamame
- ¼ cup radish, sliced
- 1 large Hass avocado, peeled, pitted, sliced
- 1 nori sheet, crumbled
- 2 tsp. roasted sesame seeds
- 1 tsp. salt

Instructions:

1. Bring a medium-sized pot filled halfway with water to a boil over medium-high heat.
2. Add the sugar snaps and cook them for about 2 minutes.
3. Remove from heat, drain excess water, transfer the sugar snaps to a medium-sized bowl and set aside for now.
4. Fill the pot with water again, add the teaspoon of salt and bring to a boil over medium-high heat.
5. Add edamame and let them cook for about 6 minutes.

6. Remove from heat, drain excess water, transfer the soybeans to the bowl with sugar snaps and let them cool down for about 5 minutes.

7. Combine all ingredients, except the nori crumbs and roasted sesame seeds, in a medium-sized bowl.

8. Carefully stir, using a spoon until all ingredients are evenly coated in oil.

9. Top the salad with the nori crumbs and roasted sesame seeds.

10. Transfer the bowl to the fridge and allow the salad to cool for at least 30 minutes.

11. Serve chilled and enjoy!

Nutritional Value Per Serving:

Calories 409

Carbohydrates 7 g

Fats 38.25 g

Protein 7.6 g

Flourless Bread

Prep time: 5 minutes

Cook time: 35 minutes

Serves: 12

Ingredients:

- 1 tsp. coconut oil
- 6 tbsp. water
- 2 tbsp. flaxseed, ground
- 1 cup almond butter
- 1 cup pumpkin
- 1 ½ tsp. baking powder
- ½ tsp. cinnamon
- 1 cup organic soy protein, vanilla flavor
- ¼ cup pumpkin seeds, raw or roasted
- ½ tsp. nutmeg

Instructions:

1. Preheat the oven to 320°F.
2. Use a parchment paper to line a large loaf pan and grease the paper with the coconut oil.
3. Combine flax seeds with water in a small bowl. Allow the seeds to soak for about 10 minutes.
4. After 10 minutes, put all the ingredients except the roasted pumpkin seeds in a blender or food processor. If desired, include the optional nutmeg.

Pulse until a smooth batter is formed, scraping the sides of the blender or food processor if necessary.

5. Move the batter into the pan and allow the mixture to sit for a few minutes.

6. Place the pan in the oven and bake for 20 minutes. Remove the bread and top it with the pumpkin seeds, then bake for another 15-20 minutes, or until a knife comes out clean.

7. Allow a few minutes to cool the bread.

8. Slice the bread into 12 slices.

9. Serve warm or cold and enjoy!

Nutritional Value Per Serving:

Calories 191

Carbohydrates 6 g

Fats 14.7 g

Protein 10.8 g

Walnut & Mushroom Loaf

Prep time: 5 hours

Serves: 10

Ingredients:

- 2 tbsp. coconut oil
- 2 cups walnuts
- 3 portobello mushroom caps, stems removed
- ½ cup green onion, sliced
- 2 cups fresh baby spinach leaves

Marinade:

- 1 tbsp. balsamic vinegar
- 1 tbsp. soy sauce
- 1 tsp. cumin
- Pinch of Himalayan salt

Instructions:

1. Grease a large cheese mold or loaf pan that fits in a dehydrator with coconut oil and set it aside.
2. In a medium-sized bowl, cover the walnuts with water and soak them for at least 8 hours. Rinse and drain the walnuts after soaking, and make sure no water is left.

3. Mix the marinade ingredients until no lumps remain.

4. Cut the portobello mushroom caps into small pieces. Add to the marinade bowl and stir until all pieces are evenly coated. Set the mushrooms aside for 30 minutes.

5. After 30 minutes, put the walnuts into a food processor or blender and pulse into tiny bits. Add the marinated mushroom pieces and green onion and continue pulsing the ingredients into a smooth mixture with tiny chunks. This should take about 2 minutes.

6. Transfer the mixture into the cheese mold and sprinkle with some additional salt.

7. Cover the mold with parchment paper and place the walnut and mushroom loaf into a dehydrator. Dehydrate the loaf at 90°F for about 2 hours.

8. After 2 hours, flip the mold upside down and dehydrate for another 2 hours.

9. Take the loaf out of the mold and cut it into 10 slices or chunks.

10. Serve each slice with a handful of baby spinach leaves and enjoy!

Nutritional Value Per Serving:

Calories 195

Carbohydrates 7 g

Fats 18.25 g

Protein 4.5 g

Savory Coconut Pancake

Prep time: 12 minutes

Cook time: 2 minutes

Serves: 1

Ingredients:

- ¼ cup coconut flour
- ¼ cup water
- ¼ cup green onion, diced
- 1 tbsp. flax seeds, ground
- ¼ tsp. baking powder
- ¼ tsp. turmeric
- Sea salt and black pepper to taste
- 1 tsp. coconut oil
- A handful of fresh rocket

Instructions:

1. In a medium-sized bowl, mix all the ingredients except the coconut oil and rocket together until no lumps remain. Set aside for up to 5 minutes.

2. Put a medium-sized skillet over medium-low heat and add the coconut oil.

3. As the oil shimmers, pour in the coconut flour mixture and allow the pancake to firm up.

4. Flip the pancake carefully by loosening the edges with a spatula, then cover the skillet with a plate,

turning the skillet upside down, and sliding the pancake back into the skillet.

5. Cook the pancake for another 2 minutes. If desired, add seasonings to taste.

6. Serve the coconut pancake warm, garnished with a handful of rocket, and enjoy!

Nutritional Value Per Serving:

Calories 281

Carbohydrates 9 g

Fats 22.05 g

Protein 8.2 g

Spicy Satay Tofu Salad

Prep time: 8 minutes

Cook time: 18 minutes

Serves: 2

Ingredients:

- 1 (12 oz. pack) extra-firm tofu, drained and cubed
- ¼ cup peanut butter
- ½ tbsp. smoked paprika
- 1 tbsp. sesame oil
- ¼ tbsp. red chili flakes
- 2 drops liquid smoke
- 2 tbsp. water
- 1 tbsp. black sesame seeds

Salad:

- 4 cups fresh baby spinach leaves, rinsed, drained
- ¼ cup fresh mint leaves, chopped
- 2 tbsp. lemon juice
- 2 tbsp. avocado oil
- ¼ cup roasted cashews, unsalted

Instructions:

1. Preheat oven to 395°F and use a parchment paper to line a baking tray.

2. Put the peanut butter, paprika, sesame oil, chili flakes, and liquid smoke into a large bowl.

3. Add the water to the bowl and mix thoroughly until all the ingredients are combined.

4. Put the tofu cubes in the bowl with the peanut butter mixture and stir gently until all cubes are evenly covered.

5. Transfer the covered tofu cubes onto the baking tray, spread them out evenly, and sprinkle the sesame seeds over them.

6. Bake the tofu cubes in the oven for about 20 minutes, or until browned and firm.

7. In a bowl, mix the salad ingredients together.

8. Take the tofu out of the oven and let the cubes cool for about 2 minutes.

9. Divide the salad and serve the tofu on top enjoy!

Nutritional Value Per Serving:

Calories 656.1

Carbohydrates 5 g

Fats 54.4 g

Protein 29 g

Lemon Rosemary Almond Slices

Prep time: 5 minutes

Cook time: 20 minutes

Serves: 4

Ingredients:

- 1 (12 oz. pack) extra-firm tofu, drained
- 1 cup full-fat coconut milk
- 1 cup almond flour

Crust:

- ½ cup raw almonds
- 1 sprig rosemary leaves, stems removed
- 1 tbsp. organic lemon zest
- 1 tsp. Himalayan salt
- 1 garlic clove, minced
- 1 tsp. ground black pepper

Instructions:

1. Preheat the oven to 395°F and use a parchment paper to line a baking tray.
2. Press the tofu down on a plate to get rid of any excess water and cut the block into 8 slices. Set the slices aside.
3. Put the almonds and rosemary into a food processor and process until chunky.

4. For the remaining ingredients, add them to the food processor and blend until thoroughly combined.
5. Transfer mixture to a bowl. Pour the coconut milk into another medium-sized bowl and put the almond flour in a third medium bowl.
6. Take a slice of tofu, dip each side in the bowl with almond flour and shake off any excess.
7. Dip the slice of flour-covered tofu into the coconut milk, and finally, dip it into the bowl with the lemon rosemary crust mix.
8. Place the coated slice of tofu onto the baking tray and repeat the process for all the tofu slices. Make sure to leave sufficient space between each slice.
9. Put the tray in the oven and bake the tofu slices for about 20 minutes, until crispy.
10. Allow the slices cool down for about a minute.
11. Serve with a light salad of greens as a side dish and enjoy!

Nutritional Value Per Serving:

Calories 542

Carbohydrates 6 g

Fats 38.4 g

Protein 17.9 g

Sausage bread

Prep time: 4 hours

Servings: 8

Difficulty:

Ingredients:

- 1 ½ teaspoons dry yeast
- 3 cups flour
- 1 teaspoon sugar
- 1 ½ teaspoons salt
- 1 1/3 cups whey
- 1 tablespoon oil
- 1 cup chopped smoked sausage

Instructions:

1. Fold all the ingredients in the order that is recommended specifically for your model.
2. Set the required parameters for baking bread.
3. When ready, remove the delicious hot bread.
4. Wait for it to cool down and enjoy with sausage.

Nutritional Value Per Serving:

Calories 234

Carbohydrates 4 g

Fats 5.1 g

Protein 7.4 g

Cheese sausage bread

Prep time: 4 hours

Servings: 8

Difficulty:

Ingredients:

- 1 teaspoon dry yeast
- 3 ½ cups flour
- 1 teaspoon salt
- 1 tablespoon sugar
- 1 ½ tablespoons oil
- 2 tablespoons smoked sausage
- 2 tablespoons grated cheese
- 1 tablespoon chopped garlic
- 1 cup water

Instructions:

1. Cut the sausage into small cubes.
2. Grate the cheese on a grater; chop the garlic.
3. Add the ingredients to the bread machine according to the instructions.
4. Turn on the baking program and let it do the work.

Nutritional Value Per Serving:

Carbohydrates 4 g

Calories 260

Fats 5.6 g

Protein 7.7 g

Bread with Beef

Prep time: 2 hours

Servings: 6

Difficulty:

Ingredients:

- 5 oz beef
- 15 oz almond flour
- 5 oz rye flour
- 1 onion
- 3 teaspoons dry yeast
- 5 tablespoons olive oil
- 1 tablespoon sugar
- Sea salt
- ground black pepper

Instructions:

1. Pour the warm water into the 15 oz of the wheat flour and rye flour and leave overnight.
2. Chop the onions and cut the beef into cubes.
3. Fry the onions until clear and golden brown and then mix in the bacon and fry on low heat for 20 minutes until soft.
4. Combine the yeast with the warm water, mixing until smooth consistency and then combine the

yeast with the flour, salt, and sugar, but don't forget to mix and knead well.

5. Add in the fried onions with the beef and black pepper and mix well.

6. Pour some oil into a bread machine and place the dough into the bread maker. Cover the dough with the towel and leave for 1 hour.

7. Close the lid and turn the bread machine on the basic/white bread program.

8. Bake the bread until the medium crust, and after the bread is ready to take it out and leave for 1 hour covered with the towel, and only then you can slice the bread.

Nutritional Value Per Serving:

Carbohydrates 6 g

Fats 21 g

Protein 13 g

Calories 499

Hazelnut honey bread

Prep time: 3 hours 10 minutes

Servings: 10

Difficulty:

Ingredients:

- ½ cup lukewarm milk
- 2 teaspoons butter, melted and cooled
- 2 teaspoons liquid honey
- 2/3 teaspoons salt
- 1/3 cup cooked wild rice, cooled
- 1/3 cup whole grain flour
- 2/3 teaspoons caraway seeds
- 1 cup almond flour, sifted
- 1 teaspoon active dry yeast
- 1/3 cup hazelnuts, chopped

Instructions:

1. Prepare all of the ingredients for your bread and measuring means (a cup, a spoon, kitchen scales).
2. Carefully measure the ingredients into the pan, except the nuts and seeds.
3. Place all of the ingredients into the bread bucket in the right order, following the manual for your bread machine.
4. Close the cover.

5. Select the program of your bread machine to BASIC and choose the crust color to MEDIUM.
6. Press START.
7. After the signal, add the nuts and seeds into the dough.
8. Wait until the program completes.
9. When done, take the bucket out and let it cool for 5-10 minutes.
10. Shake the loaf from the pan and let cool for 30 minutes on a cooling rack.
11. Slice, serve and enjoy the taste of fragrant homemade bread.

Nutritional Value Per Serving:

Calories 113

Carbohydrates 5 g

Fats 2.8 g

Protein 3.6 g

Coconut milk bread

Prep time: 3 hours

Servings: 10

Difficulty:

Ingredients:

- 1 whole egg
- ½ cup lukewarm milk
- ½ cup lukewarm coconut milk
- ¼ cup butter, melted and cooled
- 2 tablespoons liquid honey
- 4 cups almond flour, sifted
- 1 tablespoon active dry yeast
- 1 teaspoon salt
- ½ cup coconut chips

Instructions:

1. Prepare all of the ingredients for your bread and measuring means (a cup, a spoon, kitchen scales).
2. Carefully measure the ingredients into the pan, except the coconut chips.
3. Place all of the ingredients into the bread bucket in the right order, following the manual for your bread machine.
4. Close the cover.

5. Select the program of your bread machine to SWEET and choose the crust color to MEDIUM.
6. Press START.
7. After the signal, add the coconut chips into the dough.
8. Wait until the program completes.
9. When done, take the bucket out and let it cool for 5-10 minutes.
10. Shake the loaf from the pan and let cool for 30 minutes on a cooling rack.
11. Slice, serve and enjoy the taste of fragrant homemade bread.

Nutritional Value Per Serving:

Carbohydrates 6 g

Fats 15.3 g

Protein 9.5 g

Calories 421

Tangy Green Salad

Prep time: 5 minutes

Serves: 3

Ingredients:

- 4 teaspoons white wine vinegar
- ½ cup cherry tomatoes, halved
- 2 teaspoons olive oil
- Dash pepper
- 1/8 teaspoon salt
- 2 teaspoons minced fresh basil
- 3 cups torn mixed salad greens
- ¾ teaspoon honey
- 1 tablespoon shredded Parmesan cheese

Preparation:

1. Whisk vinegar, fresh basil, olive oil, honey, salt, and dash pepper in a small bowl until blended.
2. In a separate large bowl, combine tomatoes and salad greens.
3. Drizzle with vinaigrette and sprinkle with cheese.
4. Enjoy your meal.

Nutritional Value Per Serving:

Calories 1092

Carbohydrates 15 g

Fats 86 g

Protein 57 g

Chicken Breast & Zucchini Salad

Prep time: 10 minutes

Cook time: 10 minutes

Serves: 2

Ingredients:

- ¼ cup plus 1-tablespoon olive oil
- 1-pound boneless, skinless chicken breasts
- 1 ¼ pounds zucchini, thinly sliced
- ¼ cup fresh lemon juice
- ½ red onion, thinly sliced
- Coarse salt and ground pepper
- ¾ cup chopped pecans
- 1 bunch (about 8 ounces) spinach, chopped
- ¼ cup grated Parmesan cheese
- ¼ cup chopped fresh mint

Preparation:

1. Whisk together lemon juice and ¼ cup oil then season with pepper and salt.
2. Add zucchini and toss to coat. Marinate as you cook chicken.
3. over medium heat, heat the tablespoon of oil that remained in a large nonstick skillet. Cook chicken for 8-10 minutes each side until golden brown.

Season with pepper and salt. When cooked slice thinly.

4. Toss chicken with onion, parmesan cheese, pecans, spinach, mint and zucchini mixture.

5. Enjoy your meal.

Nutritional Value Per Serving:

Calories 530

Carbohydrates 15 g

Fats 19 g

Protein 34 g

Curried Pumpkin Soup

Prep time: 5 minutes

Cook time: 6 minutes

Serves: 3

Ingredients:

- 1 (29-ounce) can pumpkin
- 3 tablespoons all-purpose flour
- 2 tablespoons butter
- 1-tablespoon white sugar
- 1 1/2 cups half-and-half cream
- 2 tablespoons curry powder
- 4 cups vegetable broth
- 2 tablespoons pumpkin seeds (optional)
- 2 tablespoons soy sauce
- Salt and pepper to taste

Preparation:

1. Preheat the oven to 375 degrees F.
2. Set pumpkin seeds on a baking sheet in a layer and toast in the oven for 8-10 minutes.
3. Melt butter over medium heat in a large pot and stir in curry powder and flour until smooth.
4. While stirring, cook until mixture bubbles and then whisk in broth gradually.

5. Stir in pumpkin and half-and-half then season with salt, sugar, soy sauce, and pepper. Remove from heat and garnish with pumpkin seeds.
6. Enjoy your meal.

Nutritional Value Per Serving:

Calories 692

Carbohydrates 12 g

Fats 4 g

Protein 25 g

Beef Filled Lettuce Wraps

Prep time: 8 minutes

Cook time: 2 minutes

Serves: 2

Ingredients:

- 1-pound ground beef
- 2 teaspoons vegetable oil
- 2 scallions, chopped
- 2 -inch piece ginger, finely grated
- ¼ cup chopped peanuts
- 2 cloves garlic, minced
- 1 head lettuce leaves separated, cleaned and dried
- 1-teaspoon red pepper flakes
- ¼ cup hoisin sauce
- Salt and freshly ground black pepper
- 2 tablespoons soy sauce

Preparation:

1. Add vegetable oil in a skillet over medium-high heat and then add sauté beef. Cook until brown.
2. Stir in garlic, ginger, soy sauce, scallions, hoisin, and red pepper flakes and cook for 2 minutes. Remove from heat and add peanuts then season with pepper and salt.
3. Serve wrapped in lettuce cups.

4. Enjoy your meal.

Nutritional info:

Calories 454

Carbohydrates 16 g

Fats 7 g

Protein 47 g

Chapter 10: Dinner Recipes

Stuffed Zucchini

Prep time: 5 minutes

Cook time: 30 minutes

Serves: 2

Ingredients:

- 1 large zucchini
- 2 tbsp. olive oil
- ¼ cup green onion, chopped
- 1 garlic clove, minced
- 1 cup fresh baby spinach leaves
- A handful of fresh rocket, chopped
- Sea salt and black pepper to taste
- ¼ cup vegan cheese
- Pinch of dried parsley

Instructions:

1. Preheat oven to 380°F and use a parchment paper to line a baking tray.
2. Cut the zucchini in half lengthwise and scoop out most of the pulp.
3. Mash the zucchini pulp in a small bowl with a masher and set it aside.
4. Heat a skillet over medium heat and add half of the olive oil.

5. Add the zucchini pulp, chopped onion, and minced garlic to the skillet.
6. Stir continuously, cooking the ingredients for up to 5 minutes before adding the baby spinach and rocket.
7. Stir for a few seconds, add salt and pepper to taste, and turn off the heat.
8. Add the vegan cheese and stir well to ensure all ingredients are incorporated and the cheese has melted.
9. Scoop the mixture into the zucchini halves and transfer them onto the baking tray.
10. Cover the baking tray with aluminum foil and transfer it to the oven.
11. Bake the stuffed zucchini halves for 25 minutes. Then, turn off the oven, uncover the baking tray, and put the uncovered zucchini halves back into the oven for about 5 minutes.
12. Serve the stuffed zucchini garnished with the remaining olive oil and some dried parsley.
13. Serve and enjoy!

Nutritional Value Per Serving:

Calories 359.5

Carbohydrates 7 g

Fats 32.5 g

Protein 7.3 g

Avocado Fries

Prep time: 3 minutes

Cook time: 25 minutes

Serves: 2

Ingredients:

- 1 tbsp. olive oil
- ½ cup almond flour
- ¼ tsp. cayenne pepper
- ¼ tsp. smoked paprika
- Pinch of salt
- ¾ tbsp. unsweetened almond milk
- 1 medium Hass avocado, pitted, peeled
- 1 tsp. lime juice

Instructions:

1. Preheat the oven to 400°F.
2. Use a parchment paper to line a baking tray and grease the paper with olive oil.
3. In a small bowl, combine the flour, cayenne pepper, smoked paprika, and salt.
4. Pour the almond milk into another small bowl.
5. Slice the peeled avocado into 10 equally-sized fries.

6. Coat all sides of the fries in the flour mixture, dip in almond milk, and coat with another layer of flour.
7. Transfer the coated fries to the greased baking tray.
8. Bake the fries for 5 minutes, then flip them over and bake for another 10 minutes. Flip the fries again and bake for 5 more minutes.
9. Flip the fries one more time, sprinkle them with the lime juice, and bake them for a final 5 minutes.
10. Remove the baking tray out of the oven and allow the fries to cool down for a few minutes.
11. Serve warm with any low-carb (vegan) sauce and enjoy!

Nutritional Value Per Serving:

Calories 333.7

Carbohydrates 4 g

Fats 31.9 g

Protein 7 g

Mushroom Zoodle Pasta

Prep time: 10 minutes

Cook time: 16 minutes

Serves: 4

Ingredients:

- 3 large zucchinis
- ½ tsp. salt
- 1 tbsp. coconut oil
- 1 large green onion, diced
- 3 garlic cloves, minced
- 5 cups oyster mushrooms, chopped
- Pinch each of nutmeg, onion powder, paprika powder, white pepper, and salt
- 1 cup full-fat coconut milk
- ½ cup vegan mozzarella
- ½ cup baby spinach leaves, chopped
- ¼ cup fresh thyme, chopped
- 1 tbsp. miso paste

Instructions:

1. In a large bowl, toss the zoodles or zucchini slices with half a teaspoon of salt and set aside.
2. Add coconut oil in a large skillet, over medium heat, and add the coconut oil.

3. Add the onion and cook until translucent, for about 5 minutes while stirring occasionally.

4. Stir in the minced garlic, chopped mushrooms, and remaining seasonings.

5. Cook all ingredients in the skillet for about 3 minutes, stirring continuously.

6. Reduce heat to medium-low and slowly incorporate the coconut milk, followed by the mozzarella.

7. Cover the skillet and let the ingredients heat through for about 8 minutes, stirring occasionally.

8. Drain any excess liquid from the salted zoodles by dabbing them with paper towels.

9. Add the dry zoodles to the skillet with the chopped spinach and stir well until all ingredients are combined.

10. Turn off the heat and top the mushroom zoodle pasta with the chopped thyme.

11. Add more seasonings to taste, serve the pasta in a bowl, and enjoy!

Nutritional Value Per Serving:

Calories 421.6

Carbohydrates 13 g

Fats 34.9 g

Protein 11.5 g

Quick Veggie Protein Bowl

Prep time: 5 minutes

Cook time: 13 minutes

Serves: 1

Ingredients:

- 4 oz. extra-firm tofu, drained
- ¼ tsp. turmeric
- ¼ tsp. cayenne pepper
- 1 tbsp. coconut oil
- 1 cup broccoli florets, diced
- 1 cup Chinese kale, diced
- ½ cup button mushrooms, diced
- ½ tsp. dried oregano
- Himalayan salt
- Black pepper to taste
- ½ tsp. paprika
- ¼ cup of fresh oregano, diced

Instructions:

1. Cut the tofu into tiny pieces and season with the turmeric and cayenne pepper.
2. Warm a large skillet and add ¾ of the coconut oil.
3. Once oil is heated, add the tofu and cook it for about 5 minutes, stirring continuously.

4. Transfer the cooked tofu to a medium-sized bowl and set it aside.

5. Add the remaining coconut oil, diced broccoli florets, Chinese kale, button mushrooms, and the remaining herbs to the skillet. Use paprika, pepper, and salt to taste.

6. Cook the vegetables for 6-8 minutes, stirring continuously.

7. Transfer the cooked veggies and tofu to the bowl. Garnish with the optional fresh oregano.

8. Serve and enjoy!

Nutritional Value Per Serving:

Calories 596

Carbohydrates 6 g

Fats 20.95 g

Protein 17.8 g

Vizza

Prep time: minutes

Cook time: minutes

Serves:

Ingredients:
Crust:

- 16 oz. cauliflower rice
- 3 flax eggs
- 2 tbsp. chia seeds
- ½ cup almond flour
- ½ tsp. garlic powder
- ½ tsp. dried basil
- Pinch of salt
- 2 tsp. water

Topping:

- ½ cup simple marinara sauce
- 1 medium zucchini, sliced
- 1 medium green bell pepper, pitted, cored, sliced
- 1 cup button mushrooms, diced
- ½ cup vegan cheese
- Sea salt
- Black pepper, ground
- 1 jalapeño pepper, pitted, cored, diced
- pinch of cayenne pepper

- A handful of fresh rockets

Instructions:

1. Preheat oven to 395°F and use a parchment paper to line a baking tray.

2. Transfer the cauliflower rice to a large saucepan and add enough water to cover the 'rice.' Over medium heat, bring the water to a soft boil. Cover the saucepan, turn down the heat to medium-low, and allow the rice to simmer for about 5 minutes before draining the water off. This step can be skipped if store-bought cauliflower rice is used.

3. Transfer the cauliflower rice onto a clean dish towel and close the cloth by holding the edges. Wring out any excess water by twisting the lower part of the towel that contains the rice.

4. Once the cauliflower rice is completely drained, transfer the towel to the freezer for up to 15 minutes. Doing so will cool the rice.

5. When the cauliflower rice has cooled completely, put it into a large bowl.

6. Add the flax eggs, chia seeds, almond flour, garlic, dried basil, and salt. Combine all the ingredients into a firm, kneadable dough. If the dough is too firm, add the optional 2 tablespoons of water.

7. Spread the dough over the baking dish's surface entire. The uncooked crust should be about ¼-inch thick.

8. Bake the crust in the oven for 25 minutes, then sprinkle some additional water on top and bake for another 5 minutes. The top of the crust will turn lightly golden.

9. Allow the crust to cool for a few minutes.

10. Spread the marinara sauce evenly over the golden crust. Do the same for the vegetables.

11. Finally, garnish the vizza with vegan cheese, optional jalapeño, and cayenne pepper.

12. Season the vizza with salt and pepper and transfer it back into the oven for a few more minutes.

13. Serve the vizza warm, garnished with a handful of fresh rocket, and enjoy!

Nutritional Value Per Serving:

Calories 360.9

Carbohydrates 8 g

Fats 28.85 g

Protein 13.5 g

Tofu Cheese Nuggets & Zucchini Fries

Prep time: 5 minutes

Cook time: 18 minutes

Serves: 2

Ingredients:

Tofu Cheese Nuggets:

- 1 (12 oz. pack) extra-firm tofu, drained, cubed
- ½ cup smoked chipotle cream cheese
- ½ cup almond flour
- 2 tbsp. water

Zucchini Fries:

- 2 tsp. red chili flakes
- ½ cup almond flour
- ¼ cup olive oil
- 1 large zucchini, skinned

Instructions:

1. Preheat oven to 395°F and use a parchment paper to line a baking tray.
2. Put the cream cheese, ½ cup almond flour, and water into a large bowl and mix thoroughly until all the ingredients are combined.
3. Add in tofu cubes and coat all the cubes evenly.

4. Transfer the coated tofu cubes onto one half of the baking tray and set it aside.
5. Put the chili flakes and almond flour into a large bowl and mix until all ingredients are combined.
6. Pour the olive oil into a medium-sized bowl and dip each zucchini stick into the oil. Make sure to cover all fries evenly.
7. Put the zucchini fries in the bowl with the almond flour mixture and gently stir the fries around until they are all evenly covered.
8. Transfer the zucchini fries onto the baking tray with the tofu nuggets and spread them out evenly. If the nuggets and fries don't fit on the baking tray together, bake them in two batches.
9. Put the baking tray into the oven and bake the nuggets and fries for about 18 minutes, or until golden brown.
10. Allow the dish to cool down for about a minute.
11. Serve and enjoy with a light salad of greens as a side dish.

Nutritional Value Per Serving:

Calories 813.5

Carbohydrates 7 g

Fats 72.1 g

Protein 30.35 g

Avocado Spring Rolls

Prep time: 20 minutes

Cook time: 1 minute

Serves: 4

Ingredients:

- 2 medium Hass avocados, peeled, pitted, sliced
- 1-inch piece ginger, grated
- 1 garlic clove, minced
- Juice of ½ lemon
- ½ cup cabbage, shredded
- ¼ cup carrots, julienned or matchsticks
- 4-6 coconut wraps
- 2 tbsp. olive oil

Spicy Almond Sauce:

- ½ cup almond butter
- 2 tsp. low-sodium soy sauce
- ½ tsp. rice vinegar
- Juice of ½ lemon
- ½ tsp. chili garlic paste
- 1 tbsp. low-carb maple syrup
- 2 tsp. sesame oil

Instructions:

1. Gently toss together the sliced avocado, ginger, garlic, lemon juice, cabbage, and julienned carrots in a small bowl.
2. Put a coconut wrap on a flat and dry surface. Place about ¼ of the avocado mixture in the center of the wrap.
3. Fold the wrap about ½ inch inward on two parallel sides and roll the wrap up until the mixture is covered.
4. Repeat with the remaining 3-5 wraps until all of the avocado mixture is used.
5. Put a skillet over medium-high heat and warm the olive oil until shimmering.
6. Add the spring rolls to the skillet and brown them, about 30 seconds on each side.
7. Put all the sauce ingredients into a medium-sized bowl and stir thoroughly. Add one or more tablespoons of warm water, if necessary, to achieve the desired consistency.
8. Serve the spring rolls warm with the spicy almond sauce as a dip and enjoy!

Nutritional Value Per Serving:

Calories 503
Carbohydrates 11 g
Fats 45 g
Protein 10 g

Cauliflower Curry Soup

Prep time: 5 minutes

Cook time: 40 minutes

Serves: 4

Ingredients:

- 1 large cauliflower, chopped
- 4 tbsp. olive oil
- ½ red onion, finely chopped
- 4 garlic cloves, minced
- 1 tbsp. yellow curry paste
- 1-inch piece ginger, grated
- 1 (12 oz. pack) extra-firm tofu, drained, scrambled
- 1 tsp. chili flakes
- Juice of 1 medium lime
- 4 cups vegetable broth
- 1 tbsp. sesame oil
- 1 tsp. low-sodium soy sauce
- 1 cup full-fat coconut milk

Instructions:

1. Preheat oven to 395°F and use a parchment paper to line a baking tray.
2. Put the cauliflower florets on the baking tray and drizzle 2 tablespoons of olive oil over them, covering them evenly.

3. Put the baking tray into the oven and bake for about 25-30 minutes, until the florets are golden brown.
4. Add the 2 tablespoons that remained of olive oil to a skillet over medium heat.
5. Remove the oven and put it aside for a few minutes to let the cauliflower florets cool down.
6. Add garlic and onion to the skillet and fry for about a minute, stirring occasionally.
7. Add the curry paste to the pot along with the ginger, scrambled tofu, and chili flakes. Stir for another minute.
8. Put the baked cauliflower florets into a blender or food processor, along with the vegetable broth, sesame oil, soy sauce, and coconut milk.
9. Blend these ingredients until smooth, then transfer the mixture into the pot.
10. Incorporate all the ingredients, occasionally stirring until the contents of the pot start to cook. Once the soup reaches the boiling point, bring the heat down to a simmer.
11. Cover and allow about 10 minutes to simmer. Take the pot the heat and set aside to cool for a few minutes.
12. Enjoy!

Nutritional Value Per Serving:

Calories 390.5 g

Carbohydrates 6 g

Fats 34.2 g

Protein 12.25 g

Crispy Tofu Burgers

Prep time: 5 minutes

Cook time: 20 minutes

Serves: 8

Ingredients:

- 10 oz. pack, drained extra-firm tofu
- 1 minced clove garlic
- ½ cup coconut milk
- 2 tbsp. soy sauce
- ¼ cup sesame oil
- 2 tbsp. rice vinegar
- 1 cup coconut flour

Crust:

- 1 tsp. chili flakes
- ¼ cup nori flakes
- ½ cup crushed cashews
- ½ cup sesame seeds

Instructions:

1. Preheat oven to 390°F and use a parchment paper to line on a baking tray.
2. Drain excess water from the tofu by press it on a plate. Slice into 8 and set aside.
3. Combine garlic, soy sauce, rice vinegar, coconut oil, and sesame oil in a medium-sized bowl.

4. In a different bowl, mix all ingredients of the crust.
5. In a third different bowl, add coconut flour and dip a tofu slice in the flour. To remove excess flour, shake it off.
6. Immerse the tofu in the mixture with coconut and then immerse it into the crust mix.
7. Put the tofu on the baking tray and repeat the process for the remainder of the tofu.
8. Space the tofus while on the baking tray.
9. Add the tofus to the oven and bake for 10 minutes on each side, or until crispy and brown.
10. Allow 2 minutes to cool before serving alongside a green salad.

Nutritional Value Per Serving:

Calories 321

Carbohydrates 4 g

Fats 27.9 g

Protein 10.7 g

Avocado Chocolate Pudding

Prep time: 10 minutes

Serves: 4

Ingredients:

- 4 peeled and pitted Hass avocados, sliced
- 2 teaspoons vanilla extract
- 1 teaspoon cinnamon powder
- 1 teaspoon stevia sweetener
- ¼ cup crushed dark chocolate
- 4 tablespoons unsweetened cocoa powder
- 2 cups fresh mint leaves
- 2 teaspoons lemon zest
- ¼ teaspoon salt
- 2 tsp. lemon juice
- ¼ cup coconut milk

Instructions:

1. Add all required ingredients, including the optional lemon juice and zest to a food processor or blender. Blend to combine everything.
2. Scoop the pudding into a bowl and cover.
3. Put in a fridge for a minimum of 8 hours.
4. Top with mint leaves when serving!

Nutritional Value Per Serving:

Calories 371

Carbohydrates 8 g

Fats 33 g   Protein 7.4 g

Fatty Chocolate Bombs

Prep time: 40 minutes

Serves: 12

Ingredients:

- ¼ cup organic soy protein, chocolate flavor
- ½ cup coconut butter
- ¼ cup coconut oil
- ½ tsp. stevia powder
- pinch of salt
- a few fresh mint leaves

Instructions:

1. Line a small square cake tin with parchment paper and set it aside.
2. In a medium-sized bowl, use a mixer to combine all the ingredients, including the optional salt and chopped mint leaves. Make sure all ingredients are incorporated, and no lumps remain in the batter.
3. Pour the mixture into the prepared tin.
4. Transfer the cake tin to the freezer and allow the mixture to sit for about 30 minutes.
5. Once set, take out the cake tin and remove the chocolate chunk. Cut it into 12 squares.
6. Serve the fatty chocolate bombs with more optional mint leaves on top and enjoy!

Nutritional Value Per Serving:

Calories 115

Carbohydrates 2 g

Fats 11.7 g

Protein 1.25 g

Zucchini noodles Alfredo

Prep time: 10 minutes

Cook time: 15 minutes

Serves: 4

Ingredients:

- 3 zucchinis, medium in size
- 2 cloves of garlic, minced
- ¾ cup parmesan cheese, grated
- ½ cup almond milk, unsweetened
- 1/3 cup heavy cream
- 1 tablespoon arrowroot powder
- ¼ teaspoon nutmeg
- 1 teaspoon butter
- black pepper to taste.

Instructions:

1. Use a spiralizer to make zucchini noodles.
2. In a skillet, heat up the butter over medium heat.
3. Add garlic into the skillet and cook for a minute.
4. Minimize heat to low. Add almond milk, nutmeg & heavy cream and stir. (let it simmer)
5. In a bowl, add the arrowroot and 2 tablespoons of water. Whisk to dissolve it, making certain that there aren't any lumps. Add the mixture together with parmesan cheese into the skillet and skillet.

6. Add in the black pepper and stir till the cheese melts.
7. Omit the sauce from the pan and set it aside.
8. Add the zoodles in the pan after patting them dry with paper towels. Stir fry for about 4 minutes.
9. Add in the sauce and stir.
10. Garnish with parsley and more parmesan cheese.

Nutritional Value Per Serving:

Calories 209

Carbohydrates 6 g

Fats 16 g

Protein 11 g

Shirataki noodles (with mushrooms)

Prep time: 10 minutes

Cook time: 15 minutes

Serves: 2

Ingredients:

- Shirataki noodles, 2 packages
- 3 cups assorted mushrooms
- Olive oil
- 2 tablespoons butter
- 2 cloves garlic
- Dried parsley, pinch
- 300ml thick cream
- 1 teaspoon almond flour
- ¼ teaspoon pepper
- ¼ teaspoon salt
- Freshly chopped parsley

Instructions:

1. Rinse and drain the shirataki noodles.
2. Add the noodles into a pan over medium heat for 3 minutes.
3. Remove the noodles from the pan, setting it aside. Heat up butter using the same pan then add garlic.

4. Add the mushrooms in the pan and cook for about 5 minutes. Make sure that the mushrooms are fully coated before removing and setting aside.

5. With the oil residing on the pan, add the dried parsley, almond flour, cream, and stir constantly to combine.

6. Add the shirataki noodles and mushrooms back into the pan mix well & season, serve & garnish.

Nutritional Value Per Serving:

Calories 237

Carbohydrates 4 g

Fats 20 g

Protein 6 g

Butternut squash noodles.

Prep time: 10 minutes

Cook time: 15 minutes

Serves: 4

Ingredients:

- 6 cups Butternut squash noodles, spiralized
- ½ cup walnuts, chopped
- ½ cup parmesan cheese, shredded
- 2 tablespoons Carepelli Extra virgin olive oil
- 1 onion, chopped
- 2 cloves garlic, minced
- ¼ teaspoon black pepper, ground
- Salt to taste

Instructions:

1. Heat up the oil in a pan over medium heat.
2. Add the onion into the pan and cook for 4 minutes. (till it turns translucent)
3. Add in the garlic, letting it cook before stirring for 30 seconds.
4. Add in the noodles, cooking them for about 10 minutes. They tend to soften and shrink when cooked.
5. Add the walnuts and stir gently.

6. Serve with freshly chopped parsley and parmesan cheese.

Nutritional Value Per Serving:

Calories 408

Carbohydrates 6 g

Fats 7 g

Protein 5.4 g

Palmini noodles (with sausage ragu)

Prep time: 5 minutes

Cook time: 35 minutes

Serves: 4

Ingredients;

- 5 bratwurst sausages, without casings
- 2/3 cup parmesan cheese, grated
- ½ cup parsley, chopped
- ¼ cup Ruby port wine
- 28oz whole tomatoes, peeled
- 3 bay leaves
- 1 carrot, medium in size & grated
- 1 Oregano
- Palmini noodles, 1 can
- 1 tablespoon Fennel seeds
- 2 tablespoons Extra-virgin olive oil, divided
- 2 tablespoons garlic, chopped
- 1 teaspoon red pepper flakes.

Instructions:

1. Heat up I tablespoon of olive oil in a Dutch oven over medium heat. Add in the fennel seeds and bratwurst, cooking until the sausage begins browns. (takes 5 minutes)

2. Add in the carrot right away and cook with the sausage till it is entirely cooked. (another 5 minutes)
3. Add the tablespoon of olive oil that remained into the Dutch oven. Add in oregano, garlic, and red pepper flakes and cook for about 30 seconds.
4. Pour in the wine, bringing it to a boil. Cook for about 2 minutes till it almost evaporates.
5. Add in the tomatoes and bay leaves. Minimize the heat and simmer for 15 minutes. (Remove the bay leaves)
6. Add in the noodles and combine well.
7. Add in parmesan and parsley, stirring for 3 minutes.
8. Serve.

Nutritional Value Per Serving:

Calories 253

Carbohydrates 4.7 g

Fats 6 g

Protein 6.9 g

Kelp noodles (with sesame chicken)

Prep time: 5 minutes

Cook time: 25 minutes

Serves: 4

Ingredients;

- 1 lb. chicken breast, cut in pieces
- 10 oz. mushrooms, sliced
- 12 oz. kelp noodles
- 2 cup broccoli
- 3 carrots, large in size & chopped
- 1 teaspoon olive oil

Sauce ingredients;

- 2 tablespoons toasted sesame oil
- 3 tablespoon sesame seeds
- 2 cloves garlic, minced
- 1/3 cup coconut aminos.

Directions:

1. Heat 1 teaspoon of olive oil on medium-low heat in a skillet.
2. Add the mushrooms and fry for about 6 to 8 minutes. (ensure the mushroom liquid has completely evaporated)

3. Include the chicken, broccoli, and carrots. Fry for about 8 minutes.
4. In a bowl, add and whisk all the sauce ingredients.
5. Include the noodles and sauce to the pan. (cook for 5 minutes)
6. Season with sea salt.

Nutritional Value Per Serving:

Calories 394

Carbohydrates 7 g

Fats 10 g

Protein 29 g

Kelp noodle salad.

Prep time: 10 minutes

Cook time: 0 minutes

Serves: 4

Salad Ingredients;

- 3 green onions, sliced
- 1 (11oz/340g) pack kelp noodles
- 1 cucumber, julienned
- ¼ cup carrots, grated
- ½ cup cashews, crushed
- 0.5 oz. cilantro, minced

Dressing ingredients;

- 2.3oz almond butter
- 1 garlic clove, minced
- 1 tablespoon tamari
- 1 tablespoon swerve
- 2 tablespoons lime juice
- 1 teaspoon chili oil
- 1 teaspoon ginger root, grated
- 1 teaspoon sesame oil
- Red pepper flakes, pinch
- Sea salt, pinch.

Instructions:

1. In a bowl, mix the salad ingredients.
2. In a jar, mix the dressing ingredients.
3. Pour the dressing into the initial bowl.
4. Toss to mix and serve.

Nutritional Value Per Serving:

Calories 240

Carbohydrates 4.6 g

Fats 11 g

Protein 7 g

Baked spaghetti squash (with meatballs and marinara)

Prep time: 5 minutes

Cook time: 1.5 hours

Serves: 6

Spaghetti squash ingredients

- 1 tablespoon olive oil
- 1 teaspoon sea salt (Himalayan)
- 1 teaspoon pepper
- 1 large spaghetti squash

Directions

1. Begin with preheating your oven to 400F.
2. On your sheet pan, spread your parchment paper.
3. On the spaghetti squash, drizzle the olive oil. Sprinkle the salt and pepper too.
4. Place the spaghetti squash on the pan and insert it in the oven.
5. Bake for 40 minutes.
6. Take it out once it has baked and let it cool.
7. Use a fork to omit the squash into a bowl.

Meatball ingredients

- 1 pound/455g Italian sausage
- ½ pound ground beef (lean)

- 1 large carrot (chopped)
- 1 small red onion(chopped)
- 3 garlic cloves (peeled)
- 2 eggs (large)
- 2 tablespoons sun-dried tomatoes in oil (minced)
- 3 tablespoons parsley
- ¼ teaspoon red pepper (crushed)
- 1 ½ teaspoon salt
- 1 cup cannellini beans (drained & white)

Directions

1. In a food processor, place 1 chopped carrot, 1 chopped onion, 3 peeled cloves of garlic and the drained cannellini beans. Process until it becomes entirely smooth.
2. In a bowl, place the ground meat, parsley, eggs, salt, & red pepper.
3. Add the bean mixture in the bowl and thoroughly mix the contents by hand.
4. Line your baking sheet with parchment paper.
5. Shape 8 meatballs and place them on the parchment paper.
6. Bake in your oven for 30 minutes with the spaghetti squash.

Marinara ingredients

- 6 cloves, garlic, peeled
- 1 small red onion, chopped
- 2 large carrots, chopped
- ½ cup parsley, chopped
- ¼ cup basil, chopped
- ½ tablespoon balsamic vinegar
- 3 tablespoons olive oil
- 2 cans or 28-ounce crushed tomatoes
- 1 can or 14-ounces tomato sauce
- 1 teaspoon salt
- ½ teaspoon pepper.

Directions

1. In a saucepot heat 2 tablespoons of the olive oil on medium heat. Add the chopped ingredients (carrots, onion, garlic) and sauté for 5 minutes until they soften.

2. Add the remaining ingredients. (tomatoes, parsley, salt, pepper, and basil)

3. Minimize the heat and simmer until the meatballs are done. (Keep it covered) Remove the meatballs from the oven for the next step.

4. Add the meatballs and balsamic vinegar to the sauce and let it simmer for 15 minutes.

Nutritional Value Per Serving:

Calories 541

Carbs 7 g

Fiber 4 g

Fat 6 g

Low carb fettuccine Alfredo

Prep time: 5 minutes

Cook time: 30 minutes

Serves: 3

Ingredients

- 4 tablespoons butter
- 2 tablespoons minced garlic
- 2 cups heavy whipping cream
- 1 block parmesan cheese about 5 ounces (rind attached)
- Palmini heart of Palm noodles (1 can)
- Pink Himalayan salt (for taste).

Directions

1. Using a saucepan, melt the butter over medium heat.
2. Add the cream, garlic, and salt and stir.
3. Add the rind from the cheese to the mixture.
4. Grate the cheese into the saucepan and stir.
5. Allow several minutes to simmer. (till it attains the consistency you like)
6. Remove the rind and discard.
7. Drain and rinse the Palmini noodles.
8. Add the noodles to the sauce.
9. Remove from the heat and serve.

Nutritional Value Per Serving:

Calories 453

Carbohydrates 4.1 g

Fats 16 g

Protein 6.9 g

Stove made Keto Cauliflower Mac and cheese.

Prep time: 15 minutes

Cook time: 30 minutes

Serves: 4

Ingredients;

- 1 head cauliflower (separated into florets)
- 3 tablespoons butter (salted)
- 2 teaspoons arrow powder/ ½ teaspoon konjac
- ½ teaspoon Dijon mustard
- ¼ teaspoon black pepper (ground)
- ¼ teaspoon garlic powder
- 1 ½ cups cheddar cheese (shredded & sharp)
- 1 cup heavy cream
- ¼ tsp Kosher salt.

Directions:

1. Using a Dutch oven, brown the butter over medium heat. This will take about 5 minutes.
2. Add your heavy cream, mustard, garlic powder, black pepper, and salt into the Dutch oven.
3. Add in the cauliflower and stir, ensuring every piece is coated.
4. Simmer for about 15 minutes. (Till the cauliflower soften)

5. Mix the arrowroot powder/ konjac powder with a few tablespoons of water. Pour this into the Dutch oven and stir. (Till it forms a thick consistency)
6. Add your cheddar cheese and stir. Ensure it completely melts & serve.

Nutritional Value Per Serving:

Calories 323

Carbs 7 g

Protein 2 g

Fat 11 g

Peanut Butter Bombs

Prep time: 40 minutes

Serves: 20

Ingredients:

- 1 cup peanut butter
- 6 tbsp. coconut flour
- ¼ cup low-carb maple syrup
- ¼ cup organic soy protein, chocolate flavor
- pinch of salt
- 1 tbsp. water
- ¾ cup dark chocolate, 85% cocoa or higher, crushed

Instructions:

1. Use a parchment paper to line a baking tray and set it aside.
2. In a medium-sized bowl, use a mixer to combine all the ingredients except the crushed dark chocolate. If desired, add the optional pinch of salt. Ensure that there are no lumps remain in the batter. Add the optional water if the mixture is too thick – the batter should be spreadable.
3. Use your hands to form 20 balls and divide these over the surface of the baking tray.

4. Transfer the baking tray to the freezer and allow the balls to set for about 15 minutes.

5. Fill water in a small saucepan and put it over medium heat. Place a smaller, heat-resistant metal bowl in the water and put the crushed chocolate into it.

6. Melt the chocolate and leave the container in the water. Be careful to keep any water from getting in the chocolate. Make sure the chocolate doesn't boil because it will ruin the flavor.

7. Take the peanut butter bombs from the freezer and roll each ball in the molten chocolate, using two forks to help you. Put each ball back onto the tray and allow the molten chocolate to firm up. Repeat this step for every peanut butter bomb.

8. Refrigerate the bombs for 15 minutes, until the chocolate layer is completely firm.

9. Serve the peanut butter bombs and enjoy!

Nutritional Value Per Serving:

Calories 134

Carbohydrates 3 g

Fats 10.7 g

Protein 5 g

Cheesecake Cups

Prep time: 10 minutes

Cook time: 4 minutes

Serves: 12

Ingredients:

Crust:

- ½ cup pumpkin seeds, raw
- 6 tbsp. shredded coconut, unsweetened
- 3 tbsp. coconut oil
- 2 tbsp. organic soy protein, vanilla flavor
- ½ tsp. stevia powder
- Pinch of salt

Filling:

- 6 tbsp. coconut oil
- 6 tbsp. almond butter
- 6 tbsp. coconut cream
- 2 tbsp. lemon juice
- 2 tbsp. organic soy protein, vanilla flavor
- Pinch of salt
- ¼ tsp. xanthan gum
- ¼ tsp. stevia powder

Instructions:

1. Line a cupcake tin with 6 cupcake liners.

2. Heat a small frying pan over medium-high heat.

3. Add pumpkin seeds to the frying pan and occasionally stir for about 4 minutes.

4. Add the shredded coconut and stir thoroughly to toast everything evenly.

5. Take the frying pan from the heat and allow the ingredients to cool down before transferring them into a food processor or blender. Pulse the pumpkin seeds and shredded coconut into small crumbs.

6. Transfer the crumbs to a medium-sized bowl and add the remaining crust ingredients.

7. Combine all ingredients into a thick dough and divide this mixture into six equal-sized balls.

8. Put one ball into each of the cupcake liners, pressing and flattening the balls into a crust at the bottom of each cupcake liner.

9. Transfer the tin into the freezer and prepare the filling.

10. Heat a saucepan over medium heat and add the coconut oil. Once the coconut oil has melted, remove from heat.

11. Put the melted coconut oil, almond butter, coconut cream, lemon juice, organic soy protein, and a pinch of salt to the (uncleaned) food

processor or blender. Process these ingredients until well combined with a smooth and creamy texture.

12. Add the optional xanthan gum and stevia. Xanthan gum will help thicken the fat cheesecake bombs, while the stevia will add a sweeter flavor. Use slightly more or less stevia to taste.

13. Take the cupcake tin out of the freezer and top all crusts with filling. Make sure to divide the filling equally among the 6 cups with a tablespoon.

14. Transfer the tin back into the fridge until the cups are firm.

15. Serve the cheesecake cups at room temperature and enjoy!

Nutritional Value Per Serving:

Calories 217

Carbohydrates 3 g

Fats 21.2 g

Protein 4.2 g

Cashew Cocoa Bombs

Prep time: 30 minutes

Serves: 10

Ingredients:

- 1 cup coconut oil
- 1 cup almond butter
- ¼ cup coconut flour
- ¼ cup cocoa powder
- ¼ cup organic soy protein, chocolate flavor
- Pinch of salt
- 1 cup raw cashews, unsalted

Instructions:

1. Add almond butter and coconut oil to a saucepan and heat over medium heat.
2. Stir occasionally until the oil has melted and the ingredients are combined.
3. Pour the mixture into a bowl and, while the mixture is still warm, stir in the remaining ingredients except for the cashews. Make sure all ingredients are well combined.
4. Transfer the bowl into the freezer until the dough has become firm. This should take around 15 minutes.

5. Crush the cashews into small pieces by using a coffee grinder, food processor, or blender. Spread the crushed cashew bits over a large plate.

6. Make sure that the dough is firm before making the fat bombs.

7. Take 1 tablespoon of the firm dough mixture and roll it into a ball. Roll the ball in the crushed cashews and transfer it onto a baking tray or plate. Repeat this step for all 10 balls.

8. Place the baking tray in a refrigerator for a few minutes to allow the bombs to firm up.

9. Take the tray out of the fridge, serve the cashew cocoa bombs, and enjoy!

Nutritional Value Per Serving:

Calories 665

Carbohydrates 6.7 g

Fats 42.5 g

Protein 10.6 g

Cinnamon-Vanilla Bites

Prep time: 40 minutes

Serves: 20

Ingredients:

- 1 cup coconut oil
- 1 cup cocoa butter
- 6 tbsp. almond butter
- 2 tsp. cinnamon
- 1 tsp. vanilla extract
- ¼ cup organic soy protein, vanilla flavor
- 2 tbsp. water
- ½ cup dark chocolate

Instructions:

1. Use a parchment paper to line a large baking tray and set it aside.
2. In a medium-sized bowl, mix all the ingredients together. Make sure everything is incorporated, and no lumps remain in the dough. Add some additional water if the dough is too thick.
3. Make sure the dough is spreadable and transfer it onto the baking tray. Spread the mixture into a large rectangular chunk.
4. Transfer the baking tray to the freezer and allow it to sit for about 15 minutes.

5. Fill water in a small saucepan and put it over medium heat. Place a smaller, heat-resistant metal container inside the water and put the crushed chocolate into it.

6. Melt the chocolate in the bowl in the water. Be careful to keep any water from getting in the chocolate. Make sure the chocolate doesn't boil because it will ruin the flavor.

7. Cut the dough into 10 or 20 squares.

8. Dip each square into the molten chocolate with a fork. Repeat this for all the cinnamon-vanilla bites, putting each one back onto the baking tray.

9. Refrigerate the squares for about 15 minutes, until the chocolate coating has firmed up. Serve and enjoy!

Nutritional Value Per Serving:

Calories 249.5

Carbohydrates 2 g

Fats 26.2 g

Protein 2.1 g

Garlic bread

Prep time: 3 hours

Servings: 8

Difficulty:

Ingredients

- 1 cup milk
- 1/10 cup water
- 2 ¾ cups flour
- 1 tablespoon honey
- 1 teaspoon dry yeast
- 1 teaspoon salt
- 2 tablespoons butter
- 3 tablespoons fresh dill
- 5 cloves garlic, chopped

Instructions:

1. Start kneading the dough in the bread maker. Add flour, salt, yeast, milk, water, and honey. Stir well and shape the ball.

2. Choose the program for Dough, and set it for an hour and a half. The dough should increase significantly in volume.

3. Meanwhile, melt the butter and add the chopped garlic and dill into it. Divide the dough into 11-12

pieces. Roll each part into a thin loaf and spread each with the fragrant butter.

4. Fold the cakes one to the other, forming an accordion.

5. For 40 minutes, let the dough stand, and then select the Baking program. Set it for 50 minutes.

6. When ready, cool the bread on a grate and serve fresh.

Nutritional Value Per Serving:

Carbohydrates 5 g

Fats 2.3 g

Protein 6 g

Calories 212

Italian olive herb bread

Prep time: 3 ½ hours

Servings: 8

Difficulty:

Ingredients

- 1 cup water
- ½ cup olive brine
- 1 ½ tablespoons butter
- 3 tablespoons sugar
- 2 teaspoons salt
- 5 1/3 cups flour
- 2 teaspoons yeast
- 20 olives
- 1 ½ teaspoon Italian herbs

Instructions:

1. Cut the olives into slices.
2. Using instructions, add the ingredients to the bread maker.
3. Add olives after the beep.
4. Turn on the program.
5. Enjoy!

Nutritional Value Per Serving:

Carbohydrates 4.7 g

Fats 6.6 g

Protein 9.6 g

Calories 686

Onion black pepper bread

Prep time: 3 ½ hours

Servings: 8

Difficulty:

Ingredients

- 1 cup water
- 1 tablespoon butter
- 1 teaspoon salt
- 3 cups flour
- 3 tablespoons powdered milk
- 1 tablespoon sugar
- 1 ½ teaspoons onion
- ¾ teaspoon black pepper
- ¼ teaspoon garlic powder
- 2 teaspoons dry yeast

Instructions:

1. Using instructions, add the ingredients to the bread maker.
2. Spread the spices in a dispenser.
3. Turn on the baking program.
4. Enjoy!

Nutritional Value Per Serving:

Carbohydrates 3 g

Fats 2 g

Protein 6 g

Calories 203

Cumin bread

Prep time: 3 ½ hours

Servings: 8

Difficulty:

Ingredients

- 5 1/3 cups flour
- 1 ½ teaspoons salt
- 1 ½ tablespoons sugar
- 1 tablespoon dry yeast
- 1 ¾ cups water
- 2 tablespoons cumin
- 3 tablespoons sunflower oil

Instructions:

1. Pour warm water into the bucket of the bread maker.
2. Add salt, sugar, and sunflower oil.
3. Sift the almond flour. Pour the sifted flour into the bread maker. Add the yeast.
4. Mix the dough. If the dough turns hard, the bread will turn dense, so add a little water. If the dough turns out too soft, the bread will crumble, so add a little flour. With a wooden spatula, remove the dough from the walls of the bucket.

5. The bread maker can only be opened for the first five minutes and after a signal is sounded to add the herbs. After the signal, add two tablespoons of black cumin.

6. When the program is completed, put the bread on a grate to cool. Bon Appetit!

Nutritional Value Per Serving:

Carbohydrates 3.1 g

Fats 0.7 g

Protein 9.5 g

Calories 368

Mozzarella oregano bread

Prep time: 3 ½ hours
Servings: 8
Difficulty:

Ingredients

- 1 cup milk + egg
- ½ cup Mozzarella cheese
- 2 ¼ cups flour
- ¾ cup flour whole-grain
- 2 tablespoons sugar
- 1 teaspoon salt
- 2 teaspoons oregano
- 1 ½ teaspoons dry yeast

Instructions:

1. Using instructions, add the ingredients to the bread maker.
2. Turn on the program.
3. After the end, leave to cool on the grate.
4. Enjoy!

Nutritional Value Per Serving:

Carbohydrates 4.8 g
Fats 2.1 g
Protein 7.7 g
Calories 209

Italian raisin rosemary bread

Prep time: 3 ½ hours

Servings: 8

Difficulty:

Ingredients

- 2 eggs
- ¾ cup water
- 1 teaspoon dry yeast
- 3 cups almond flour
- 1 teaspoon salt
- 3 tablespoons rosemary, freshly chopped
- 1 tablespoon sugar
- 4 tablespoons olive oil
- 1 cup raisins
- small sprigs of rosemary for decoration

Instructions:

1. Beat the eggs in a dish and then top with water.
2. Put all the ingredients except the raisins in the bread maker in the manner indicated on its instructions.
3. Add the chopped rosemary after the flour.
4. Put the form in the bread maker and turn on the main baking program with the addition of raisins.

Add raisins at the signal, or in the middle of the batch cycle.

5. Before baking, spread the sprigs of rosemary on the surface.
6. After baking, remove the bread from the mold and allow it to cool.

Nutritional Value Per Serving:

Carbohydrates 5 g

Fats 8.8 g

Protein 7 g

Calories 312

Chapter 11: Snacks Recipes

Vegan Papaya Mousse

Prep time: 2 hours

Serves: 6

Ingredients:

- 250 grams Ripe Papaya, peeled, deseeded, and diced
- 1-2 tbsp Stevia
- a pinch of Powdered Cardamom
- 1.5 cups Coconut Cream
- ¼ cup tbsp Chia Seeds
- 50 grams Chopped Pecans

Instructions:

1. Combine papaya, stevia, and cardamom in a food processor or blender. Process until smooth.
2. Combine papaya puree, coconut cream, and chia seeds in a bowl. Stir to combine.
3. Divide mousse into serving containers and chill for at least 2 hours.
4. Serve with chopped nuts or dried fruit on top.

Nutritional Value Per Serving:

Calories 274

Carbohydrates 9 g

Fats 27 g

Protein 13 g

Sugar and Cinnamon Mug cake

Prep time: 1 minute

Cook time: 3 minutes

Serves: 1

Ingredients:

- 3 tbsp Soy Protein Powder
- 1 tsp Baking Powder
- 3 tbsp Coconut Flour
- ½ tsp Cinnamon Powder
- 1 tbsp Erythritol
- ¼ cup Coconut Milk
- ½ tsp Vanilla Extract

Instructions:

1. Combine all ingredients in a microwave-safe mug. Mix until blended well. To get a cake batter consistency, adjust milk and flour accordingly.
2. Microwave for 2 minutes in 30-second intervals.
3. Sprinkle with more cinnamon on top before serving.

Nutritional Value Per Serving:

Calories 161

Carbohydrates 8 g

Fats 14 g

Protein 2 g

Vegan Crème Brulee

Prep time: 1 hour

Cook time: 5 minutes

Serves: 6

Ingredients:

- 1 cup Almond Milk
- 1.5 cups Coconut Milk
- 1/3 cup Erythritol
- ¼ cup Cornstarch
- 1 tbsp Vanilla Extract
- 2 tsp Orange Zest

Instructions:

1. Add all the ingredients to a pot and whisk on medium heat.
2. Constantly stir until thick.
3. Scoop into ramekins and allow a minimum of one hour to chill.
4. Drizzle sugar on top and caramelize with a kitchen torch.

Nutritional Value Per Serving:

Calories 386

Carbohydrates 9 g

Fats 16 g

Protein 3 g

Dairy-Free Avocado and Mint Ice Cream

Prep time: 8 hours

Serves: 4

Ingredients:

- 1 Large Avocado, peeled and pitted
- 400 ml Coconut Milk
- 1 tbsp Vanilla Extract
- 1 tbsp Coconut Oil
- 2 tsp Powdered Stevia
- 1 cup Ice Cubes
- ¼ cup Fresh Mint Leaves
- 1 tbsp Lime Juice

Instructions:

1. Add avocados, coconut milk, vanilla extract, coconut oil, powdered stevia, lime juice, and mint leaves. Blend until smooth.
2. Put in a freezer-safe dish and freeze for 2-3 hours.
3. Take out of the freezer and stir to break up ice crystals.
4. Return to the freezer until fully set.

Nutritional Value Per Serving:

Calories 421

Carbohydrates 5 g

Fats 11 g

Protein 1 g

Piña Colada Cupcakes

Prep time: 10 minutes

Cook time: 20 minutes

Serves: 6

Ingredients:

- 1.5 cups Almond Flour
- ½ cup Erythritol
- ¼ tsp Salt
- 2 tsp Baking Powder
- 1/3 cup Coconut Oil
- 1 tbsp Ground Flax Seeds
- ½ cup Coconut Milk
- 1 tsp Rum Extract or Vanilla Extract
- ¼ cup Crushed Pineapple
- ½ cup Desiccated Coconut toasted slightly

Instructions:

1. Whisk together the flour, erythritol, salt, flax meal, and baking powder in a bowl.
2. Stir in coconut milk, rum extract, and coconut oil.
3. Fold in crushed pineapple and desiccated coconut.
4. Divide the batter into cupcake liners, filling each about 2/3 of the way.
5. Bake for 20 minutes at 375ºF.

Nutritional Value Per Serving:

Calories 397

Carbohydrates 8 g

Fats 28 g

Protein 5 g

Almond-Chia Doughnut Holes

Prep time: 4 hours

Serves: 8

Ingredients:

- 1.5 cup Walnuts
- 1 cup Dates
- ½ cup Almond Flour
- 2 tablespoons Chia Seeds

For the Glaze

- 1 tsp Vanilla Extract
- ¼ cup Coconut Oil

Instructions:

1. Mix almond flour, walnuts, dates, and chia seeds in a blender. Process until the texture is fine.
2. Divide the mixture and roll into packed balls. Put in a freezer for a minimum of 2 hours.
3. Whisk vanilla extract and coconut oil together.
4. Immerse the balls into the glaze and let them chill for up to 10 minutes and serve.

Nutritional Value Per Serving:

Calories 186

Carbohydrates 9 g

Fats 16 g

Protein 3 g

Vegan Banana Bread

Prep time: 10 minutes

Cook time: 1 hour

Serves: 12

Ingredients:

- 2 cups Almond Flour
- ¼ cup Coconut Flour
- 1 tbsp Baking Powder
- 1 tbsp Cinnamon Powder
- ¼ tsp Salt
- ¼ cup Chopped Pecans
- ½ cup Coconut Oil
- ½ cup Erythritol
- 4 Flax Eggs
- ¼ cup Almond Milk
- 1 tbsp Banana Extract

Instructions:

1. Preheat oven to 350°F.
2. Add all ingredients to a blender. Process on high until smooth.
3. Put the batter into a parchment-lined loaf pan. Top with chopped pecans.
4. Bake for 50-60 minutes.
5. Allow cooling before slicing.

Nutritional Value Per Serving:

Calories 192

Carbohydrates 6 g

Fats 18 g

Protein 3 g

Bulgogi-Spiced Tofu Wraps

Prep time: 2 hours

Cook time: 5 minutes

Serves: 6

Ingredients:
- 400 g Firm Tofu
- 200 grams Iceberg Lettuce for wrapping

For the Marinade
- 50g chopped Leeks
- 2 tbsp Soy Sauce
- 1 tsp Erythritol
- 2 tbsp Sesame Oil

For the Slaw
- 50 g White Radish, julienne
- 50 g Cucumber, julienne
- 50 g Carrots, julienne
- 20 g Scallions, julienne

For the Dip:
- 1 tbsp ml Light Soy sauce
- 2 tbsp ml Sesame oil
- 1 tsp Erythritol
- 1 tbsp Gochujang

Instructions:

1. Mix all tofu marinade ingredients in a bowl.
2. Slice the tofu into 1 inch thick cuts and marinate for not less than 2 hours.
3. While marinating, prepare the slaw. Whisk all ingredients for the dressing. Toss in all chopped vegetables. Cover and refrigerate.
4. Grill the tofu and cut into approximately 1"x3" strips.
5. Toss chopped tofu with the prepared slaw.
6. Serve with lettuce leaves for wrapping.
7. Allow cooling before slicing.

Nutritional Value Per Serving:

Calories 498

Carbohydrates 7 g

Fats 15 g

Protein 12 g

Vegan Baked Jelly Doughnuts

Prep time: 1.5 hours

Cook time: 10 minutes

Serves: 12

Ingredients:

- 1 tbsp Yeast
- 2 tbsp Warm Water
- 180 ml Soymilk
- 1 tbsp Erythritol Maple Syrup
- 1 g Baking Soda
- ¼ tsp Salt
- 1 tbsp Flaxseed Meal
- 3 tbsp Water
- 2 tbsp Olive Oil
- 500 g Almond Flour
- 150 g Desiccated Coconut
- Sugar-Free Fruit Jelly(for filling)

Instructions:

1. Drizzle yeast over warm water and allow 5 minutes to bloom.
2. Stir flaxseed meal in water and bloom for 5 minutes.
3. In a large bowl, mix together yeast mixture, flaxseed mixture, soymilk, erythritol, and olive oil.

4. Whisk almond flour and baking soda in a separate bowl. Gradually beat flour into the wet ingredients.
5. Knead the resulting dough for about 5 minutes or until smooth and elastic.
6. Place the dough in a lightly oiled bowl and cover. Allow it about 1 hour to rise in a warm place.
7. Turn the dough onto a floured surface. Roll out into ½" thickness and cut into circles.
8. Transfer to a sheet pan, cover, and leave again to rise for another hour.
9. Bake for 8-10 minutes at 420°F.
10. Place on a rack to cool.
11. Fill each doughnut with your choice of jelly using a pastry injector.
12. Coat with desiccated coconut.

Nutritional Value Per Serving:

Calories 251

Carbohydrates 9 g

Fats 22 g

Protein 9 g

Moutabelle with Keto Flatbread

Prep time: 20 minutes

Cook time: 20 minutes

Serves: 6

Ingredients:
For the Moutabelle

- 500 grams Eggplant
- 75 grams White Onion
- 10 grams Flat Parsley
- 2 tbsp tahini paste
- 2 tbsp Lemon Juice
- ¼ cup Olive Oil
- Salt, to taste
- Pepper, to taste

For the Flatbread:

- ½ cup Almond Flour
- 2 tbsp Psyllium Husk
- ¼ tsp Baking Soda
- pinch of Salt
- 1 tbsp Olive Oil
- 1 cup Lukewarm Water

Instructions:
Prepare the Flatbread:

1. Whisk together baking soda, psyllium husk, salt, and almond flour in a bowl.
2. Add in the water and olive oil.
3. Knead to form a smooth dough.
4. Leave to rest for about 15 minutes.
5. Divide the dough into 6 equal-sized parts.
6. Roll each part to a ball, then flatten with a rolling pin in between sheets of parchment paper.
7. Refrigerate until ready to use.
8. To cook, heat in a non-stick pan for 2-3 minutes per side.

Prepare the moutabelle :
1. Split each eggplant in half lengthwise. Use salt to season and brush with olive oil.
2. Grill over high heat until fully cooked. Set aside until cool enough to handle.
3. Peel the grilled eggplants, and transfer the flesh to a blender or food processor. Add in the ingredients that remained and process until smooth. You may add a little warm water if it is too thick to process.

Nutritional Value Per Serving:
Calories 371
Carbohydrates 9 g
Fats 15 g
Protein 2 g

Curry-Spiked Vegetable Latkes

Prep time: 15 minutes

Cook time: 6 minutes

Serves: 6

Ingredients:

- 100 grams Carrots, spiralized
- 100 grams Zucchini, spiralized
- 100 grams Cauliflower, minced
- 50 grams White Onion, minced
- 5 grams Parsley, chopped
- ¼ cup Almond Flour
- 1 tbsp Flax Seeds, soaked in 2 tbsp Water
- 2 tsp Curry Powder
- ½ tsp Salt
- 2 tbsp Olive Oil plus more for frying

Instructions:

1. Mix shredded vegetables, onions, parsley, almond flour, egg, salt, and curry powder in a bowl.
2. Heat olive oil in a non-stick skillet.
3. Add in the vegetable mixture, shaping each latke with an egg ring.
4. Fry each side for about 3 minutes.
5. Drain on paper towels.

Nutritional Value Per Serving:

Calories 123

Carbohydrates 5 g

Fats 12 g

Protein 2 g

Vegan Cheese Fondue

Prep time: 5 minutes

Cook time: 20 minutes

Serves: 4

Ingredients:

- 70 grams Raw Cashews
- 1 tbsp Nutritional Yeast
- 2 tsp Cider Vinegar
- 2 tbsp Gelatin
- 1 tsp Garlic Powder
- 1 tbsp Turmeric Powder
- 1 tsp Salt
- 1.5 cups Water
- 200 grams Zucchini, cut into sticks

Instructions:

1. Boil cashews for 15 minutes.
2. Process cashews, salt, yeast, vinegar, gelatin, water, turmeric powder, and garlic powder in a blender until smooth.
3. Transfer the puree into a saucepot and boil for 3-5 minutes, stirring constantly. The mixture will lump at first. Keep stirring until smooth.
4. Serve to a fondue pot with zucchini sticks.

Nutritional Value Per Serving:

Calories 126

Carbohydrates 9 g

Fats 8 g

Protein 6 g

Chocolate Peanut Butter Cookies

Prep time: 20 minutes

Cook time: 10 minutes

Serves: 14

Ingredients:

- ½ cup Peanut Butter, melted
- 3 tbsp Coconut Oil
- ½ cup Erythritol
- ½ cup Coconut Milk
- 1 tsp Vanilla Extract
- 2 cups Almond Flour
- ½ tsp Baking Soda
- ½ tsp Salt
- ½ cup Vegan Semi-Sweet Chocolate Chips

Instructions:

1. Stir together peanut butter, coconut oil, erythritol, coconut milk, and vanilla extract in a bowl.
2. Whisk salt, baking soda, and flour in a different bowl.
3. Stir the flour mixture into the mixture with oil.
4. Fold in the chocolate chips.
5. Form cookies and put them on a parchment paper-lined baking tray.
6. Bake for 10 minutes at 375°F.

Nutritional Value Per Serving:

Calories 179

Carbohydrates 5 g

Fats 16 g

Protein 5 g

Chocolate Macadamia Pralines

Prep time: 1 hour

Serves: 15

Ingredients:

- 150 grams Vegan Chocolate
- 1 tbsp Coconut Oil
- For the Filling:
- 150 grams Macadamias

Instructions:

1. In a double broiler, use coconut oil to melt chocolate.
2. Add the chocolate to praline mold. Coat every cavity evenly by swirling around.
3. Chill the mold in a chiller for about 5 minutes to allow the chocolate shells to set.
4. Remove and fill macadamias at the centers.Seal pralines with more melted chocolate, again tapping to eliminate any air bubbles.
5. Chill for five additional minutes to set completely.

Nutritional Value Per Serving:

Calories 132

Carbohydrates 7 g

Fats 11 g

Protein 2 g

Vegan Choco-Peppermint Bites

Prep time: 10 hours

Serves: 16

Ingredients:

- 1 cup Vegan Dark Chocolate Chips
- 1 cup Raw Cashews
- 8 pieces Pitted Dates, rough-chopped
- 1 tsp. Peppermint Extract
- 1 tbsp. Soy Milk
- 2 tbsp. Coconut Oil

Instructions:

1. Put cashews in a bowl with water and soak overnight.
2. Drain and put in a food processor alongside peppermint extract, coconut oil, dates, and soy milk. Process until smooth.
3. Divide the mixture into a praline mold. Use a plastic wrap to cover and freeze for at least an hour.
4. Melt chocolate chips in a double boiler.
5. Unmold the frozen cashew mixture and dip into the melted chocolate. Evenly coat and drip excess chocolate. Return to the freezer for a few minutes or until chocolate is fully set.

6. Serve chilled.

Nutritional Value Per Serving:

Calories 256

Carbohydrates 9 g

Fats 9 g

Protein 3 g

Cinnamon raisin bread

Prep time: 3 ½ hours

Servings: 8

Difficulty:

Ingredients

- 1 cup warm milk
- 2 teaspoons baker's yeast
- 1 tablespoon sugar
- 3 tablespoons butter, softened
- 3 tablespoons honey
- 1 egg
- 1 teaspoon salt
- 1 teaspoon ground cinnamon
- 3 cups almond flour
- 1 cup raisins

Instructions:

1. Soak the yeast with the sugar in warm milk for 10 minutes to allow the yeast to react.
2. Add all ingredients apart from raisins to the bread maker.
3. Choose the Basic program and run it.
4. Add the raisins at the signal. If this function is not present, add 5 minutes before the end of the batch cycle.

Nutritional Value Per Serving:

Carbohydrates 3 g

Fats 6.1 g

Protein 7.6 g

Calories 319

No-Bake Coconut Chia Macaroons

Prep time: 2 hours

Serves: 6

Ingredients:

- 1 cup Shredded Coconut
- 2 tbsp Chia Seeds
- ½ cup Coconut Cream
- ½ cup Erythritol

Instructions:

1. Combine all ingredients in a bowl. Mix until well combined.
2. Chill for about 200-30 minutes.
3. Once set, scoop the mixture into serving portions and roll into balls.
4. Return to the chiller for another hour.

Nutritional Value Per Serving:

Calories 129

Carbohydrates 5 g

Fats 12 g

Protein 2 g

Avocado Lassi

Prep time: 1 hour

Serves: 3

Ingredients:

- 1 Avocado
- 1 cup Coconut Milk
- 2 cups Ice Cubes
- 2 tbsp Erythritol
- ½ tsp Powdered Cardamom
- 1 tbsp Vanilla Extract

Instructions:

1. Combine all ingredients in a bowl. Mix until well combined.
2. Press the mixture into a rectangular silicone mold and freeze for an hour to set.
3. Slice for serving.

Nutritional Value Per Serving:

Calories 305

Carbohydrates 9 g

Fats 29 g

Protein 3 g

Vegan Fudge Revel Bars

Prep time: 1 hour

Serves: 12

Ingredients:

- 1 cup Almond Flour
- ¾ cup Erythritol
- ¾ cup Peanut Butter
- 1 tbsp Vanilla extract
- ½ cup Sugar-Free Chocolate Chips
- 2 tbsp Margarine

Instructions:

1. Mix together almond butter, coconut flour, erythritol, and vanilla extract in a bowl until well combined.
2. Press the mixture into a rectangular silicone mold and freeze for an hour to set.
3. Melt the chocolate chips with the margarine for 1-2 minutes in the microwave.
4. Pour melted chocolate on top of the mold and chill for another hour to set.
5. Slice for serving.

Nutritional Value Per Serving:

Calories 160

Carbohydrates 5 g

Fats 14 g

Protein 5 g

Chapter 12: Keto Shopping List

Strawberries	Avocado oil	Nutritional
Coconut wraps	Cauliflower rice	Yeast
Flax seeds	Walnuts	Olive oil
Maple syrup	Chipotle chili	Spinach
Pineapple	Spaghetti	Shirataki
Fresh dill	squash	noodles
Pitted Dates	Jalapeno	Sesame oil
Olive brine	pepper	Rice vinegar
Italian herbs	Onions	Garlic cloves
Cornstarch	Cumin	Ginger
Orange Zest	Salt	Sodium soy
Cheddar cheese	Tomatoes	sauce
Crushed cashews	Lime juice	Red pickled
Mandarin	Red pepper	cabbage
segments	Chickpea	Carrots
Erythritol	powder	Coconut cream
Cannellini beans	Garlic powder	Silk tofu
Desiccated	Baking powder	Ice cubes
Coconut	Chili flakes	Raspberries
Cinnamon	Chia seeds	Acai powder
powder	Hemp hearts	Soy protein
Rosewater	Sweetener	powder
Tea	Coconut milk	Hazelnut butter
Nutmeg powder	Vanilla extract	Banana essence
Powdered cloves	Virgin coconut	Quinoa
	oil	Instant coffee

Portobella mushrooms	Almond milk	Kale
Tomato paste	Vanilla essence	Truffle parmesan cheese
Panko	Coconut flour	
Paprika powder	Almond meal	Dijon mustard
Dried sage	Applesauce	Lemon juice
Black pepper	Almond flour	Chili-garlic paste
Firm tofu	Avocado	Red curry paste
Tamari	Matcha powder	Cane sugar
Sunflower oil	Baking soda	Kaffir lime leaves
Turmeric powder	Cashew butter	Coconut flakes
Broccoli	Red miso paste	Shredded mozzarella cheese
Textured-vegetable protein	Organic orange zest	
	Eggs	Plain gelatin
Red kidney beans	Wheat gluten	Italian seasoning
	Xanthan gum	Soy flour
Bell pepper	Apple cider vinegar	Chicken breast
Dried oregano	Parmesan cheese	Psyllium husk
Cocoa powder	Lemon zest	Old bay seasoning
Cacao nibs	Nutmeg	
Cilantro	Handful fresh rocket	Rosemary leaves
Zucchini		Sausage
Basil	Peanut butter	Stevia sweetener
Pine nuts	Smoked paprika	Dark chocolate
Cherry tomatoes	Liquid smoke	Fresh mint leaves

Cauliflower florets	Whey	Arrowroot powder
Vegan cheese	Milk	Ruby port wine
Nori sheets	Honey	Bay leaves
Cucumber	Whole grain flour	Noodles
Asparagus spears	Caraway seeds	Fennel seeds
Enoki mushrooms	Scallions	Coconut aminos
Capers	Lettice leaves	Swerve
Sugar snap peas	Red pepper flakes	Chili oil
Edamame	Hoisin sauce	Ginger root
Radish	Dried parsley	Papaya
Balsamic vinegar	Cayenne pepper	Powdered Cardamom
Cumin	Miso paste	Pecans
Himalayan salt	Banana Extract	California Dates
Sugar	Leeks	Vegan Semi-Sweet Chocolate Chips
Beef	Sugar-Free Fruit Jelly	Macadamias
Rye flour	Soymilk	Peppermint Extract
Coconut chips	Tahini paste	Raisins
teaspoons white wine vinegar	Eggplant	Margarine
Dash pepper	Thyme	Curry powder
Torn mixed salad greens	Pumpkin seeds	All-purpose flour
	Vegetable broth	Pumpkin

Chapter 13: Keto Frequently Asked Questions

IS THE KETOGENIC DIET SAFE?

The ketogenic diet is safe when it is done with medical or nutritional monitoring and not on its own. At first, it can cause some symptoms such as dizziness, tiredness, among others, which will disappear over the weeks. The body feels these effects from drastically reduced carbohydrates but adapts to dietary change over time.

IS IT WORTH THE KETOGENIC DIET?

The ketogenic diet is worthwhile for both epilepsy control, diabetes control, and obesity treatment since this diet has been very positive. However, as said, it needs to be done with professional monitoring, as it is a restrictive diet and causes some symptoms at first, so it cannot be done on its own.

WHAT IS KETOSIS?

As we have seen, ketosis or ketogenesis is a process where the body breaks down stored fat molecules to use them as an energy source. This breakdown generates products such as free fatty acids and glycerol that give rise to new compounds called ketone bodies. It is these compounds that form the fatty acids that will be used as a source of energy for the body.

AM I LOSING MUSCLE?

You may lose a little muscle on a diet. However, high intake of protein and high levels of ketone can help reduce muscle loss, particularly if you are lifting weights.

IS KETOGENIC DIET GOOD TO BUILD MUSCLE?

Yes, but it is not best like when on a moderate carb diet.

IS REPLENISHMENT OR CARBOHYDRATE LOADING A MUST?

No. But, a few days richer in calories can be beneficial from time to time.

WHAT IF I'M CONTINUOUSLY TIRED OR WEAK?

You cannot be in full ketosis or be using fats and ketones effectively. To counter this, decrease your intake of carbs. A supplement such as ketones or MCT oil can also help.

WHY DOES MY URINE SMELL FRUITY?

Do not worry. It is as a result of by-product excretion created during the ketosis process.

WHAT CAN I DO WHEN MY BREATH SMELLS?

Try sugar-free chewing gum or drink naturally flavored water.

WHAT CAN I DO WHEN I HAVE PROBLEMS WITH DIARRHEA AND DIGESTION?

This side effect is common, and it occurs mainly after 3-4 weeks. Just in case it persists, you should consume more vegetables with high fiber.

Conclusion

Thank you for making it through to the end of this book. I hope it was informative and able to provide you with all of the tools you need to achieve your goals.

You now have all you need to get started with a ketogenic diet. It is a great way to lose weight. With some little changes in your eating habits, you will be well on your way to losing those pounds you have struggled with for a long time.

Finally, if you found this book helpful and insightful for your journey, please leave a short review on Amazon. It means a lot to me!

Thanks for your support and happy Keto journey!!

Legal & Disclaimer

The information in this book is designed not to replace any kind of professional or medical advice; it is also not meant to take place of the need to have independent legal, financial, medical, or other advice that is, as needed. This book contains information for educational and entertainment purposes only.

Upon using the contents and information contained in this book, you agree to hold harmless the Author from and against any damages, costs, and expenses, including any legal fees potentially resulting from the application of any of the information provided by this book. This disclaimer applies to any loss, damages or injury caused by the use and application, whether directly or indirectly, of any advice or information presented, whether for breach of contract, tort, negligence, personal injury, criminal intent, or under any other cause of action.

You agree to accept all risks of using the information presented inside this book.

By reading this book, you agree to consult an expert (attorney, doctor, dietician or any other as you may need) prior to applying the information, techniques, and remedies in this guide book.

CPSIA information can be obtained
at www.ICGtesting.com
Printed in the USA
BVHW090851150221
600147BV00012B/1258